MW01170308

CONTENTS

Introduction

Which Blender Should You Use?

Blenders have come a long way in recent years, the level of power has significantly increased and the price tag reduced. This means you can blend a variety of fruits, vegetables, nuts and seeds in a convenient and cost effective manner.

The recipes in this book are aimed at all high power blenders. I personally have and use the Nutri Ninja Pro Blender (BL450) on a daily basis. But I know that these recipes can be used just as effectively in the Nutribullet. Both blenders are very similar in terms of what they can blend.

What This Book Can Do For You

You will find a selection of healthy yet delicious recipes to inspire you to make consuming raw fruit and vegetables a part of your daily diet. Each section will come with some helpful tips and hints, together with a breakdown of the nutritional attributes of each recipe.

The Basics of Smoothie Making

Of course you purchased this book for recipe inspiration. However, it doesn't hurt to have an idea of the basics of smoothie making, and to know what combinations work well together.

There may be some ingredients in my recipes that you can either not get hold of where you live, or you really cannot stomach. For me, I have a mainly dislike relationship with celery. No matter how much I try and disguise it in a smoothie, it just keeps on shining through. So, instead of trying to force myself to drink it, I will just swap it out with something else.

Hopefully this guide will give you the confidence to play around with the recipes and experiment with some of your own creations.

If you loosely follow these pointers, you won't go far wrong.

The Smoothie Base Liquid

Depending on the ingredients you are using, most smoothies will require a liquid of some sort to make them a consistency that is pleasant to drink.

Water

I normally use water, mainly because I always have it in the house. Of course, water is fantastic for staying adequately hydrated and much cheaper than buying up lots of other liquids to blend. Be careful how much you add, if you add too much it will take away some of the taste of the smoothie.

Coconut Water

My second go to liquid base is coconut water. You may well have seen it taking up more shelf space at the local supermarket as the health benefits are becoming more well known.

Not only does it taste great, it is also packed full of nutrients. In fact, coconut water contains magnesium, calcium, potassium, sodium and phosphorus. The five essential electrolytes found in the human body. The fat content of coconut water is very low, meaning you can drink it in the knowledge that not only is it doing you good, it is also not making you pile on the pounds.

Unsweetened Almond Milk

Almond milk is 100% plant based and rich in antioxidants. It is a great source of vitamin E which contributes to the protection of cells from oxidative stress. Not only that, almond milk is naturally low in fat and easy to digest due to it being naturally lactose free. The smooth, creamy and nutty taste will add to the taste of any smoothie.

As long as you use an almond milk that is unsweetened with no additives, it will be low in carbohydrates, meaning that by using it you won't significantly increase your blood sugar levels. Other benefits include being low in sodium with no cholesterol or saturated fat. It is high in the healthy fats, including omega fatty acids.

Almond milk is high in fibre, aiding the digestion of your smoothie.

Vitamins include iron and riboflavin which are necessary for muscle growth and healing.

Although almond milk only contains 1 gram of protein per serving, it contains plenty of B vitamins such as iron and riboflavin, both important for muscle growth and healing.

Chilled Green Tea

You can't have missed the hype surrounding the health benefits of green tea. And it is with good reason. It is rich in polyphenols and catechins that can help fight various cancers and help your heart function properly.

High Fibre Carbohydrates

When people talk about carbohydrates we often think of bread, pasta, potatoes etc. However, carbohydrates can be found in many plant-based foods. Carbohydrates often hit the headlines when diet and health is being discussed. They are frequently given a bad rap for making you put on weight.

However, if you are eating the right kinds of carbs they will provide you with plenty of health benefits and play a vital role in reaching your optimum health levels.

Not all carbohydrates are created equally, so swapping out the unhealthy unnatural ones for unprocessed or minimally processed plant-based foods, will provide you with essential fibres which may help protect you against a number of health conditions. These fibre rich carbohydrates will also leave you with a fuller feeling, meaning you aren't constantly craving snacks that might not be quite so good for you.

There are many high fibre carbohydrates that are good for you, some of which you will find in the following recipes. They include spinach, cucumber, kale, celery, apples, raspberries, blueberries, strawberries.

The Fruits and Vegetables

As I mention a few times in this book, the best ingredients you can put in your smoothie are the green leafy variety. Spinach, kale, romaine lettuce, watercress, whatever you have available. Even if you don't enjoy these and think they will ruin your smoothie, please give them a try. Start off with a little and gradually build up. As you taste buds adjust you will want to include more, especially once you begin to notice the health benefits of consuming them.

When picking which fruits and vegetables to use, a great rule of thumb is to go colourful. Experiment with produce that is red, green, purple, orange and yellow. If you are able, freeze some of your fruits and vegetables. Chopped bananas, pineapple, melon, berries, grapes and other exotic fruits are great to just grab out of the freezer and pop in your blender.

Many of the smoothie recipes in this book are suitable for freezing and turning into ice lollies. The perfect nutrient rich and healthy pudding, that actually tastes good.

Healthy Fats

By adding some healthy fats to your smoothie you will fill fuller for longer, feel more energized and benefit from the extra nutrients and vitamins included in those ingredients.

What healthy fats can you include? My favourite that I like to use is avocado. Adding avocado will make the smoothie quite a bit thicker so you may want to add more liquid. If you don't like the taste of avocados very much you can easily mask it with some raspberries, strawberries or a ripe banana.

Avocados are incredibly nutritious and come with many health benefits. They are very high in potassium (more so than a banana). Avocados are incredibly high in monounsaturated oleic acid, a "heart healthy" fatty acid that is believed to be one of the main reasons for the health benefits of olive oil. Avocados also have a lot of fibre in them which as we know is great for filling fuller. It will also benefit our digestive system.

Nuts and seeds are another brilliant addition to a smoothie. In particular, as the Nutri Ninja (and the Nutri bullet if you are using one instead) is such a powerful machine, they can be blended up to a very smooth consistency, which for some people means they are easier to consume.

Most of us don't eat nearly enough seeds and nuts. They are incredibly healthy and are packed full of fibre, fat, protein, minerals and vitamins.

The best way to decide which nuts and seeds to eat is to eat a variety of them. Many supermarkets and health shops sell mixed bags so you can throw a handful of these into a smoothie.

Nuts I like to include are almonds, brazil nuts, almonds, walnuts, pecans and cashews.

For seeds I tend to use a mix of sesame, flax, sunflower, pumpkin and chia.

Each of these nuts and seeds bring an amazing amount of health benefits and I really encourage you to try and add some to your smoothies.

This is my favourite one. Chocolate. High quality dark chocolate has been proven in scientific studies to be a great antioxidant, and rich in healthy fats. Try and choose an organic one that is high in cocoa content (70-90%). You will find some yummy recipes which include dark chocolate.

Proteins

By adding protein rich ingredients to your smoothies you will help curb your hunger pangs as well as aid tissue repair, build lean muscle (which helps you burn more fat,) and provide you with more energy.

You may choose to get your proteins from a manufactured powder which you simply stir into your smoothie. I don't use protein powders so couldn't comment on which ones are better than others, I just try to use natural ingredients from foods to get my protein intake.

Here are some of my preferred protein sources to use in smoothies;

Unsweetened almond milk, coconut milk, flax seeds, oats, chia seeds, soya milk. There are of course many more and it depends on your tastes and what is available locally for you.

Why Drink Smoothies?

Do you feel tired, overweight or simply have no zest for life? The old saying of we are what we eat, has never been more true. The Western world is facing unprecedented levels of obesity, diabetes and other serious health problems.

You can do something about it. And the good news? It doesn't have to be hard. You don't (and shouldn't) need to deprive yourself of food to be healthy. It is perfectly ok to eat enough food to feel full, as long as it is the right kind of food. The other goods news; it doesn't have to turn your life upside down. You can add as little as one smoothie a day, and combined with other healthy eating choices you will soon begin to see the differences.

Drinking Smoothies for Improved Health

We all know that the best solution for good health is prevention. Unfortunately this isn't always possible. We all go through periods of our lives when we are not taking good enough care of our bodies. Or perhaps you are, and you've just been unlucky and developed an ailment despite your best intentions. Whatever the reason, by drinking at least a smoothie a day, you can help alleviate your problem and give your body the best chance of fighting the problem.

Smoothies are a fantastic choice for staying hydrated. Fruits and vegetables contain large amounts of water. The human body is made up of roughly 60 per cent water and we need to make sure we stay well hydrated, especially if you are active.

Smoothies for Weight Loss

Yes, smoothies can be used to aid you in weight loss. But it is important to make sure you are drinking the right combination to ensure that you are not denying your body of the vitals nutrients for full health. I go in to more details in the chapter dedicated to weight loss, suggesting how you might lose weight and improve your health with the right selection of ingredients.

Using your Nutri Ninja Blender

Using your blender is fairly straight forward, which is the beauty of it. However, it is worth being aware of a few basics so that you can use your blender to its full potential and avoid any pitfalls.

You can prepare a wide array of wholesome recipes, including smoothies, sauces, soups and meals. Although this book purely focuses on smoothies, future books will cover the other types of recipes. The variety of different food types you can use is what makes this blender so versatile.

Order of Ingredients

It is important to put the easier to blend items in first followed by the harder to blend items. So, for example, in our Green Machine Smoothie recipe you would put the spinach in first, followed by avocado, cucumber, pineapple and then finally the ice cubes. Then top up with your liquid. This way when you connect the cup to the blade section the ice cubes are at the bottom by the blades, making it easier to blend to a smooth consistency.

What Can I Put In?

You can put most things in the blender without the need to take out the pips or seeds, with the exception of the following;

Apples seeds, apricot stones, cherry stones, plum stones, peach stones, avocado stones.

Once you have been through a few of our recipes and are feeling a bit more confident, you can experiment with different ingredients and measurements. There are no strict rules on what you put with what, other than what your taste buds might think of it! As a basic rule of thumb though, I would follow these combination guidelines;

50% Leafy Greens - Kale, Spinach, Spring Greens, Romaine Lettuce, Swiss Chard

50% Fruit

Optional Boost - I like to add an extra nutrient boost to my smoothies, these can be; Seeds, nuts, ground flaxseed, goji berries, acai berries etc

Liquid - Fill the Nutri Ninja cup to the max line with a liquid of your choice (water, coconut water, unsweetened nut milks, soya milk etc)

Using Frozen Ingredients

Where we can, we tend to use frozen fruits. Especially blueberries, strawberries, pineapple, mango and bananas. Not only does this mean we can use them year round, it also means we don't need to add extra ice cubes. If you don't or can't get the frozen variety, you can chop them up as soon as you have bought them and store them in bags in the freezer. Of course if you would prefer to just use them as you buy them fresh, just pop in some ice cubes to get a nice smooth and cold drink. Due to the amazing power of the Nutri Ninja Blender, you can easily blend ice cubes and any frozen fruits and vegetables.

How Thick Do You Like Your Smoothie?

Depending on how you like the consistency of your smoothie you may want to adjust the recipes slightly. The following ingredients will make your drink thicker or thinner so you can get it tasting just how you like it;

Thinner

Water

Coconut water

Green Tea (chilled)

Unsweetened nut milks

Thicker

Avocado

Ripe banana

Chia Seeds

Oatmeal

Making it Sweet

If you are used to drinking sweeter smoothies it may take a while to adjust your taste buds. To make it easier on yourself why not try adding some of the following sugar alternatives. It is really important not to add refined sugar. The less processed a sugar is, the better it is for you.

Raw honey

Dried fruits such as dates, dried figs, raisins and apricots

Maple syrup (natural)

We mainly add honey when we feel like a bit of extra sweetness in our smoothies.

TIP: Don't overfill the cup. Don't go past the marked out max line, this may result in you breaking the seal and the smoothie leaking in the future.

Blending It

Once all your chosen ingredients are in the cup, screw the blade part on to the cup and fix it to the motor part of the Nutri Ninja. This is where the Nutri Ninja is a game changer for us. It will blend your ingredients into a really smooth drink, no chunks or seedy bits floating around.

It shouldn't need more than 30 seconds of blending to get the desired consistency. If you want to, you can drink it straight from the cup. Or pour some out into a glass and store the rest in the fridge by putting the supplied lid on top.

Should You Buy Organic Food?

Once upon a time everything was eaten in season and grown in naturally fertilized soils. Now, as we all know, fields are sprayed with pesticides, herbicides and fungicides. The demand for out of season fruits and vegetables has meant that products are often picked before they are ripe so that they can be transported to reach the supermarket shelves in all corners of the world. By which time much of the nutritional value has dramatically reduced.

Buying organic produce is always the better option. Due to the sustainable way in which it is grown, without pesticides, preservatives or artificial ingredients. However, it isn't always possible to buy organic, whether it is due to financial reasons (it is more expensive) or it simply isn't readily available where you live. Where possible, I try to use local organic produce. Of course this is not always feasible, and in these cases I will use the next best thing. For example, if I want to add blueberries and they are not in season, I will buy some frozen blueberries. In fact, frozen fruits are fantastic to put in smoothies. A cold smoothie tastes yummy and the convenience of just grabbing it out of the freezer will mean you make and consume way more smoothies.

If you are only able to buy a few organic items then the following are the ones you should make priority;

Apples

Strawberries

Grapes

Celery

Peaches

Spinach

Cucumbers

Kale

Pineapples

Soft Citrus

Carrots

If you are unsure of the origin always follow these guidelines;

Peel non organic hard fruits and vegetables before blending or wash very thoroughly.

Wash all berries before blending.

Remove skins of citrus fruits that may have been waxed.

Tips for a Healthy Lifestyle

Stay Hydrated

Try to drink at least 8 glasses of water each day. If you drink a glass when you think you are hungry this will help determine if you are really hungry or just dehydrated. Drinking more water can help speed up your metabolism. Water helps blood transport oxygen and other important nutrients around your body. Water will help you when you work out, not only to stay hydrated, but to keep your joints lubricated. Drinking water can also help keep your skin hydrated and younger looking. Flushing out all those toxins can only be a good think for creating your outer glow!

Keep a Food Journal

By keeping a daily food diary you can see the times of day when you are slipping into bad habits. For example, I know that the evenings are a hard time for me. I am used to snacking whilst I'm writing or watching a film. Pre-empt this time by preparing a smoothie or healthy snack in advance.

Healthy Snacks on Standby

Keep healthy quick bites nearby. A handful of seeds and nuts or some raw carrots or cucumber to dip into some yummy hummus. Carry some fruit with you when you are out and about so you are not tempted to duck into the supermarket for a quick treat.

Take Regular Exercise

Find something that *you* enjoy doing. Go for a walk, run, cycle, swim, or whatever makes you happy. Mix it up and combine a variety of exercises. Get friends and family involved, join clubs. Not only will exercise help create a healthy lifestyle physically, it will help your mind.

Go Natural

Swap the processed food for natural. The less human intervention it has had the better. Hopefully, once you have integrated a smoothie or 2 into your daily diet, you will start to lean towards the more natural foods anyway.

Eat a Balanced Diet

Make sure you are getting enough of each food. Keep them as 'clean' and natural as possible. Be sure to include lean proteins, fibre, healthy fats and good carbohydrates. Protein will help you feel full for longer periods of time. What's more, protein will help you build and keep muscle mass. Muscle naturally burns more calories than fat. So don't forget the protein! Good sources of protein include chicken, salmon, turkey and lean steak.

Get Enough Sleep

It is easy to skip on sleep. And not always through choice! We all need differing amounts of sleep but I know when I haven't had enough I am cranky, tired and reaching for the nearest energy boost. Of course, if you have unavoidably missed out on your zzz's then try and get more energy with an extra smoothie rather than junk food.

Treat Yourself

Look after yourself. Treat yourself to things that make you feel great. Whether it's a massage, a spa day, a new hair cut or a new outfit, reward yourself for improving your health. Leading a healthy lifestyle is a package, nutrition plays a huge part in it but so do other factors. Look after the whole of you.

The Recipes

The bit you are waiting for, getting stuck into making your smoothies. I have tried where possible to split the smoothie recipes into chapters according to their health benefits. Of course there is a lot of overlap between chapters, and what I recommend most of all is to switch it up each day as much as your ingredients will allow. Variety of raw food is the key to a healthy you.

Each recipe measurements are based on using the larger cup size (24oz). This cup size generally makes 2 large drinks or 3 small ones (depending on how much you want to drink of course!) If you want to make less then just reduce the recipes accordingly.

Remember, if you want to make a smoothie thinner then add some more liquid, or if you prefer a thicker consistency add ice or some extra ingredients like banana, avocado, chia seeds etc.

My measurements do not need to be followed precisely, which is why I have used 'handfuls' quite a bit throughout the recipes. Don't get too caught up in the exact quantities, use that time to get blending and drinking. Use mine as a rough guide. For example, if I say 2 handfuls of spinach and 1 handful of mixed berries, you know you need to use roughly twice the amount of spinach as berries.

A lot of the smoothie recipes include kale, spinach or another kind of leafy green. This is because greens are the powerhouse of nutrition. They are packed with proteins, antioxidants, vitamins and a variety of other benefits your body needs. Where you see a green leafy ingredient, please feel free to substitute it for what you have available. For example, if it says spinach, feel free to swap it for kale, or romaine lettuce or mixed spring greens etc. Rotate them round as much as possible so that you can gain the different nutritional benefit from each ingredient.

Most of all, enjoy creating your smoothies and reaping the rewards of a healthy new you!

Smoothie Recipes for Weight Loss

Whether you want to lose a few pounds or a lot of pounds, you will be pleased to know that smoothies can help you. Not only can you make some fabulous tasting ones, you will also fuel your body with an incredible array of nutrients, vital for a healthy lifestyle.

Many people like to know how many calories they are consuming when they are trying to lose weight. Personally I don't like to do this as it kind of takes the fun out of eating. For instance, if adding half an avocado would take me over a recommended calorie meal allowance, I certainly wouldn't leave it out. The reason being is that avocados, whilst high in fat, they are high in the fat that is incredibly good for you!

Making Smoothies a Daily Habit

In my opinion, it makes sense to start on your road to healthy and wholesome eating by making smoothie drinking a daily habit. Pick some smoothies from this book and plan your food for the week ahead. Make sure you have the necessary ingredient and write out which smoothies you are going to have and when.

If you can, make them and consume them at the same time every day. For me, this is first thing in the morning, right after I have had a glass of cold water (the best way to start the day!) Do this EVERY single day without fail. Even if you are missing an ingredient, still make it. Or you don't think you fancy a smoothie, still make it. It will make you feel amazing for the day.

After a while of drinking a healthy smoothie each day you will start to notice that you don't necessarily crave the other junk and processed food so much.

Losing Weight with Smoothies

If you want to lose weight then why not try and swap one of your meals for a smoothie? For me, this would be breakfast, I make a smoothie big enough that it will last me for a mid-morning guzzle too. Or have a smoothie for breakfast and lunch and then eat a healthy and wholesome meal at dinner time.

Only eat whole foods that have no added nasties in them. Opt for wholegrain where you can and still pile up the vegetables on your plate. If you feel hungry in the day then snack on healthy foods. Raw fruit and vegetables or boiled eggs are just a few examples.

Go Easy on Yourself

Don't feel bad if you break this and end up scoffing a bag of crisps or a pizza - just get back on track the next day if you can. Personally, I think some people need this little leeway in their diet for 'forbidden foods' - I know I certainly do! Call it a 5 or 10% allowance. Just keep it balanced. Of course if you don't have the urge for the odd slice of cake or chocolate bar then no problem, don't go forcing yourself!

Ok, let's dive into the recipes then. As with all of them, feel free to chop them around according to your tastes and what ingredients you have available.

Berry Peachy

1 handful of kale
2 peaches
2 handfuls of frozen or fresh mixed berries
1 handful (or around 12) grapes
2 tablespoons of ground flaxseeds
Water
Ice cubes

Making It

Wash all the ingredients. Chop the peaches. Put all of the ingredients in your Nutri Ninja and blend. Add water to maximum line or less if you prefer a thicker consistency.

Did You Know

Peaches are a great source of vitamins C and A. Peaches have a high water and fibre content which helps you to feel full for longer.

Ground flaxseeds contain many healthy fats and have a high fibre content. They can be added to a variety of foods, not just smoothies, try a table spoon sprinkled on cereal. Flaxseed contains a plant-based omega-3 fatty acid (linolenic acid) that helps to increase the feelings of being full.

Boost Me Up Ginger

1 carrot
1 pear
1 apple
1cm of fresh root ginger
250ml of coconut water (or plain water)
Ice cubes

Making It

Chop the apple and remove the seeds. Place all the ingredients in your blender. You may want to start off with a smaller amount of fresh root ginger if you are not use to consuming it raw in a smoothie. Build it up gradually until you are comfortable with the zingy taste. Adjust the liquid content to desired consistency.

Did You Know

Ginger can play an integral part in the weight loss process by acting as a fat burner. Ginger helps to raise your metabolism, meaning you burn more calories. It can also act as a natural appetite suppressant, making you feel fuller and less likely to overindulge.

Carrots have an abundance of health benefits. They are a low-calorie food that also provides essential dietary fibre. This is ideal for weight management as they will make you feel fuller for longer.

Apples and pears both have a high water content and high dietary fibre, again helping with making you feel full up without adding too many calories.

Needy Seedy

2 handfuls of spinach
8 frozen or fresh strawberries
1/2 frozen banana
250ml Coconut Water
2 Tbsp of Chia Seeds
Ice cubes

Making It

This makes for a great afternoon treat. Place all of the ingredients in your blender and whizz. Enjoy this delicious smoothie safe in the knowledge that it is good for you!

Did You Know

Chia Seeds are grown natively in Mexico. They were said to be the basic survival ration of the Aztecs and Mayans. Chia seeds are super healthy as they are rich in healthy omega-3 fatty acids, antioxidants, protein, calcium, fibre and various micro nutrients. Aside from being a nutritional powerhouse, chia seeds act by expanding in size when in liquid. This means, if you drink your smoothie shortly after making it, the chia seeds will expand in your stomach, meaning you will feel much fuller for much longer. Chia seeds are 40% fibre by weight, meaning they are the best source of fibre in the world. If you are consuming chia seeds outside of a smoothie, make sure you are drinking adequate liquid (water) with them.

Bananas often get a bad rap for being high in calories. So why include them in a weight loss section? Well, bananas are filling, and as they are sweet in taste, they curb any sugar cravings you might be having. I like to snack on a ripe banana if I feel like an energy boost. A medium one is only around 100 calories, that's the same as some biscuits! I know which one will work better with my waistline and keep me feeling fuller for longer!

Strawberries are said to speed up your metabolic rate by helping to promote the production of certain fat burning hormones. Aside from the amount of antioxidants that these delicious berries contain, they also have enough fibre to help with your digestion. Strawberries make for another great snacking food. I especially like them in the evening after dinner.

Green Tea Smoothie

1 handful of frozen blueberries
1 banana
1 pinch of cinnamon
200ml chilled green tea
Ice cubes

Making It

Make the required amount of green tea and allow it to chill enough to put in the Nutri Ninja. Add all the remaining ingredients and blend for 30 seconds.

Did You Know

Green tea not only has the benefit of boosting metabolism, it is also thought to reduce bad cholesterol. It makes a brilliant base to a smoothie as it is so low in calories.

Cinnamon is a great way of improving the flavour of a smoothie, especially if you are trying to mask a taste you don't like, it can also leave you feeling fuller for longer and keeps blood sugar levels more balanced.

Blueberries are rich in nutritional value and full of powerful antioxidants, vitamin C and potassium. They contain no fat and low in calories. I tend to keep blueberries frozen (I either buy them frozen or put our own home grown ones straight in the freezer once we have picked them.) Blueberries are great for your digestive system due to the insoluble fibre they contain.

Chocolate Velvet

1 handful of kale
2 chunks of grated dark Chocolate (minimum 75% cocoa content)
1 frozen banana
200ml unsweetened almond milk (or any other nut milk/soy milk)
Ice Cubes

Making It

Place all ingredients in the Nutri Ninja and blend. Enjoy.

Shhh! Don't tell anyone we've sneaked a chocolate smoothie into a weight loss chapter! Who said losing weight had to be boring? Not I. If you enjoy chocolate please don't deny yourself of it when trying to lose weight. All that will happen, is you will crave it, you will initially resist it, and then you'll go crazy and reach for the nearest bar! Well, that's me anyway.

Did You Know

If you incorporate the best kind of dark chocolate into your diet, in moderation, you will not only satisfy that chocolate urge, you'll also be treating your body to some pretty amazing antioxidants. Dark chocolate (at least 75% cocoa) is very nutritious. Quality chocolate is actually rich in fibre, iron, magnesium amongst other minerals. So go on, enjoy it!

Red Hot Chilli Smoothie

Handful of frozen strawberries
1/2 red chilli pepper
1cm of fresh root ginger
1 cup of orange juice
Juice of half a lime
Water

Making It

Carefully chop up the chilli, removing the seeds. Maybe start with a smaller bit of chilli and taste the smoothie before adding more. Try and use freshly squeezed orange juice if you can. Put all the ingredients in and blend. Add water to make desired consistency. Go with me on this one. I know a red chilli in your smoothie might not sound quite right, but trust me, it does taste pretty good.

Did You Know

Chillis are a brilliant way to speed up your metabolism. Chilli peppers raise your endorphin level, making you feel pretty great. Chili peppers also have a compound in them call capsaicin which increases energy, acts as an appetite suppressant and boosts metabolism. Sometimes I'll add a little dark chocolate into the mix - try it, it is delicious. Just remember to handle those hot ones with care. Nothing worse than rubbing your eye when you've got hot spice on it. I've been there. Ouch.

Oh, Brussels

1 handful of spinach
3 brussel sprouts
1 apple
1/4 medium pineapple
Half a lime
250ml of coconut water
Ice cubes

Making It

If you are not a fan of the controversial sprout then maybe try with just 1 to start with and work your way up. Put all the ingredients in your Nutri Ninja and blend.

Did You Know

Ok, ok, I know. Brussel sprouts. I sense a little trepidation with this one. I almost got evicted from the house today when I revealed the ingredient in this little gem. Maybe I'm a little biased as I adore brussel sprouts, but this didn't actually taste too bad. Brussel sprouts have some incredible health benefits due to their antioxidants. Not only that, if you get them when they are in season, the sweet ones taste pretty good and are low in calories. Perfect for a weight loss smoothie. At least give it a try!

Go Green

1 handful of kale
1 handful of spinach
1 banana
1 apple
1 tablespoon of ground flaxseeds
Water
Ice cubes

Making it

Place all ingredients into blender and blend until a smooth consistency. Add more water if desired.

Did You Know

Kale and spinach are popular choices when making a green smoothie. They are excellent sources of vitamin k which your body uses to help with bone development and keeping your blood healthy. By including 2 cups of raw spinach and (or) kale in your daily smoothie you will consume your recommended daily intake of vitamin K. The high levels of vitamin A in both leafy greens also help to keep your skin clear by maintaining a healthy skin cell function.

I like to make this smoothie and have it for my breakfast.

Perfect Pears

2 handfuls of mixed spring greens
1 handful of frozen or fresh mixed berries
2 pears, chopped with the skin still on.
250ml of water

Making It

Put all ingredients in your blender and blend for 30 seconds. Add more water if required.

Did You know

The skin of a pear is said to contain about half of the pear's whole dietary fibre. The skin also contains many of the antioxidants of the pear. As pears are so fibrous they can really help with weight loss whilst providing important antioxidants and flavonoids.

Berries are also a great source of fibre, alongside other health benefits. For example, raspberries contain ketones which are said to prevent an increase in overall body fat. More importantly, berries taste fantastic and can really sweeten up a smoothie.

The Raspberry Rush

2 handfuls of spinach
1 banana
1 handful of fresh or frozen raspberries
Water
Ice cubes

Making It

Place all the ingredients in your Nutri Ninja cup. I prefer to use frozen raspberries so that I can use them year round. Blend and add more water (or other liquid) as required.

Did You Know

Raspberries have a lot going for them. Not only do they taste delicious, they are also packed full to the brim with nutrients, vitamins and minerals. They are low in fat and calories, but rich in dietary fibre and antioxidants.

Tropical Treat

2 handfuls of spinach
2 carrots
1/4 chopped pineapple
1 handful of fresh or frozen mango
Water

Making It

Put all ingredients in your Nutri Ninja cup and blend.

Did You Know

Mango is a popular fruit (especially in my house!) It has some great health promoting attributes, including dietary fibre, vitamins, minerals and antioxidant compounds. Mango is rich in vitamin A and flavonoids, including beta-carotene which is great for healthy vision. The high dietary fibre content of mangoes make them a great ingredient to include in a weight loss smoothie.

The Easy Peasy

2 handfuls of romaine lettuce
2 handfuls of fresh or frozen mango
Water

Making It

Try and pick a crisp and fresh romaine lettuce to use in your smoothie. Place all ingredients into the Nutri Ninja and blend. Feel free to substitute the water for coconut water if you fancy changing it up a bit.

Did You Know

Romaine Lettuce is a great green leafy base to use in your smoothie. The flavour is quite mild in taste, making it great to use if you are trying to get used to the richer taste of other greens. Romaine lettuce contains all 9 essential amino acids, what a great nutritional boost to include in your smoothie. Romaine lettuce is high in calcium, omega-3 essential fats and has more vitamin A than a carrot! The water content of a romaine lettuce is high, making it perfect for keeping you hydrated whilst helping you lose weight. Despite not being one of the darker greens, romaine lettuce is still very rich in minerals. It is also high in iron. What's not to like?

Energy Boost Smoothies

No matter how healthy we are trying to be, we're eating all the right foods and getting more sleep, we all hit a point where we need an energy boost. For me, this is usually mid afternoon. I used to get round this with a quick caffeine boost, or half a packet of biscuits. Needless to say, the boost was short lived. Unfortunately, the detrimental effect on my health was longer lasting.

If like me, an afternoon nap is out of the question, you'll need a quick and nutritious pick me up that doesn't involve a fake junk fix.

Smoothies can be the perfect solution. Using the Nutri Ninja makes it much easier to create a energy boosting smoothie in a short amount of time. If you are out at work or elsewhere when the slump hits, make up one of the following smoothies before you leave home and take it with you.

Feel the Beet

2 handfuls of romaine lettuce
1/2 raw beetroot
1 carrot
1/2 stick of celery
Half a lemon (if unwaxed you can leave the skin on)
Water
Ice cubes

Making It

How you use the raw beetroot will come down to your personal taste. I find it quite hard to take the earthy taste of a blended beetroot so I tend to pop mine in my juicer and use the juice to put in my Nutri Ninja. However, I know many others who love the taste so just put it straight in their blender. Adding lemon or lime juice can help mask the taste if you want to blend it for convenience. Put all the ingredients in your blender and mix until you have the desired consistency.

Did You Know

Beetroot has approximately 20 times the amount of nitrates as other vegetables. The nitrate converts into nitric oxide in our bodies which helps to provide us with longer lasting energy. Beetroot widens the blood vessels allowing oxygen to flow more easily, increasing your energy and stamina levels. Beetroot is also rich in iron, an essential mineral needed for healthy blood and energy production.

Vitamin Vrrrooom

1 handful of kale
1 handful of broccoli florets (can use frozen)
1 banana
250ml of coconut water
Ice cubes

Making It

Due to the high power of the Nutri Ninja it makes for a great machine for blending broccoli. You can use frozen broccoli if you prefer, and start with a few florets if you are not used to the taste. The banana in this recipe really helps to sweeten up the taste.

Place all the ingredients into the Nutri Ninja and blend.

Did You Know

Broccoli is full of dietary fibre, great for making you feel full up and controlling your blood sugar levels, creating longer lasting energy. Broccoli is a great source of beta-carotene, calcium, vitamin C, pottasium, magnesium and vitamin Bs.

Go Bananas

2 handfuls of kale
1 apple
2 bananas
Water
Ice cubes

Making It

If you are able to use frozen bananas then it will negate the need for using ice cubes. If they are not frozen then fresh is fine. I either buy mine frozen (often as part of a mixed bag of frozen fruit) or I will chop them up and freeze them from fresh. Place all the ingredients in the Nutri Ninja and blend.

Did You Know

Bananas are the food of choice of Jamaican Olympic sprinter Yohan Blake. Apparently he scoffs 16 bananas a day! Personally, I probably wouldn't (and couldn't!) eat that many in a day, but he is right to get his energy the natural way. Bananas help to keep your blood sugar levels stable, the sucrose contain in a banana which acts more slowly than other sugars. So, you get the same energy high as you would get from a fizzy energy drink but without the crash afterwards. You'll find me on the running track.

Grape Vitality

2 handfuls of romaine lettuce
1 carrot
2 handful of grapes
1 table spoon of ground flaxseed
250ml of water

Making It

Place all the ingredients in your blender and blend until smooth. As with other ingredients you can freeze your grapes if you want and take them from the freezer as and when you need them.

Did You Know

Grapes are a great source of vitamin B1. Vitamin B1 is great for providing your body with a great energy boost. Plus, they taste great!

Plucky Peach

1 handful of spinach
2 peaches
1 handful of fresh or frozen mango
Water
Ice cubes

Making It

Place all the ingredients in your Nutri Ninja and blend. Feel free to substitute the water with coconut water or another healthy liquid (unsweetened nut milk etc.)

Did You Know

Peaches are a rich source of carbohydrates and natural sugars so great for an energy boost. If you use dried peaches they are also a great source of iron.

Oat Me Up

1 handful of romaine lettuce
1 handful of fresh or frozen mango
1 handful of oatmeal
Juice from 2 oranges
250ml coconut water
Ice cubes

Making It

Place all ingredients in the Nutri Ninja and blend. You might need to blend the ingredients for a little longer to ensure a smoother consistency with the oats. Or if you like a bit of crunch in your smoothie then blend for the usual 20-30 seconds.

Did You Know

Oatmeal is great for boosting energy. Oats are great for controlling blood sugar levels meaning your energy levels stay balanced. Oats are of course a great source of carbohydrates, perfect for your energy needs.

Sports Drinks

Whether it is before, during or after exercise it is really important to be filling your body with the right fuel. There are plenty of sports drinks available to buy, but not all are going to help your health long term. Personally, I find them quite sickly as they tend to be really sweet. I much prefer to make my own up.

The following smoothies are quick and easy to make with your blender, and will really help you perform to the best of your ability, and then aid in the recovery post exercise. I'm not promising to turn you into the next Usain Bolt, but it'll give you a fighting chance, reach for the stars right?!

The Beetroot Bolt

1 handful of kale
1 small raw beetroot (or use beetroot juice instead)
1 apple
1/4 pineapple
1/4 cucumber
Half a lime
250ml water
Ice

Making It

I mentioned this earlier in the book, the raw beetroot can either be blended or juiced, depending on your preferences (and of course if you have a juicer.) Place all the ingredients in your Nutri Ninja and blend.

Did You Know

The Power of Beetroot

When I trained for and ran my last marathon I used raw beetroot quite a bit. I even drunk it during the marathon event itself to help my body cope with the intensity of what it was going through.

According to research from Exeter University there are two marked physiological effects from beetroot juice. It contains high levels of nitrate which widens the blood vessels, reducing blood pressure and allowing more blood to flow. It cuts the amount of oxygen needed by muscles, making exercise less tiring.

"We were amazed by the effects of beetroot juice." Professor Andy Jones University of Exeter.

Beetroot juice has been one of the biggest stories in sports science after researchers at the University of Exeter found it enables people to exercise for up to 16% longer. The startling results have led to a host of athletes – from Premiership footballers to professional cyclists – looking into its potential uses.

It took some experimenting to get this smoothie tasting just right. Raw beetroot has a distinctive earthy taste to it which I really needed to figure out a way to disguise if I was going to be able to drink it mid run.

Cool as a Cucumber

1 handful of romaine lettuce
1 apple
1/2 cucumber
Half a lime
Water
Ice cubes

Making It

Put all the ingredients in your Nutri Ninja. Add water up to the max line or less if you prefer a thicker consistency.

Did You Know

The cucumber contains over 90% water, second only to the watermelon for its high water content. This makes cucumber the ideal thirst quencher for not only hot days but for use during and after working out. If you can buy organic cucumbers, even better. This way you can blend the skin, which is where high quantities of silica is found. Silica is a mineral that helps strengthen tendons, muscles, cartilage, bones, ligaments and skin.

Walnut Wonder

1 apple
1 banana1/4 cup of walnuts1 handful of fresh or frozen raspberries
250ml of coconut water
Ice cubes

Making It

Place all the ingredients in the Nutri Ninja cup and blend. The sweetness of the raspberries and banana will mask the taste for anyone that has a dislike of walnuts.

Did You Know

Walnuts contain linolenic and linolenic fatty acid, two heart healthy essential fatty acids. Walnuts are also a great source of protein, fibre and are also high in magnesium and potassium, essential electrolytes for muscle function.

Build Me Up

1 handful of spinach
1 apple
2 bananas
4 tbsp wheatgerm
250ml of unsweetened almond milk/coconut water/water
Ice cubes

Making It

Wheatgerm can be bought at all good supermarkets, health food stores or online. Place all the ingredients in your Nutri Ninja blender. Feel free to substitute the almond milk for coconut water or plain water.

Did You Know

Wheatgerm is nutrient rich. It is high in essential fatty acids, vitamin B, amino acids and vitamin E. It is a brilliant source of energy and is said to increase stamina and performance. Wheatgerm is also a great source of protein which helps to maintain healthy muscles and regulate energy levels.

Melon Madness

2 handfuls of romaine lettuce
2 cups of seedless watermelon
1 handful of fresh or frozen strawberries
Water
Ice cubes (if not using frozen ingredients)

Making It

You won't need to include as much water in this recipe due to the high water content found in watermelons. Feel free to adjust the water levels accordingly. Place all the ingredients in the Nutri Ninja and blend. This is a smoothie perfect for hot summer days.

Did You Know

Watermelons don't contain as many nutrients as other fruits but they are high in beta-carotene and vitamin c. They also contain lycopene (the same nutrient found in tomatoes.) The high water content in watermelons make them a great ingredient to include in a smoothie to sip on to rehydrate during and after a workout.

Cashew Crazy

1 apple
1 handful of cashew nuts
2 bananas
1 tsp Spirulina
Water
Ice cubes

Making It

Place all of the ingredients in your Nutri Ninja and blend. Spirulina can be bought in all good health food shops and online. It is quite an acquired taste so you may want to get yourself used to it by starting with tiny amounts. It will also turn your smoothie a striking green colour.

Did You Know

Cashews contain monounsaturated fats which help promote good cardiovascular health. They are also great for great looking skin and hair.

Spirulina is often used by athletes as a nutritional supplement. Spirulina is a blue green algae that's been around for some 3 billion years. Spirulina is said to help protect athletes from the effects of overtraining and can help improve endurance. Spirulina helps the body to burn fat rather than carbs when working out, this allows the body to work out for longer as energy levels are kept higher.

Powered By...

2 handfuls of mixed greens (kale, spinach, romaine lettuce and any others you have)
1/2 avocado
1 handful of fresh or frozen raspberries
250ml of coconut water
Ice cubes

Making It

Get the benefits of all the greens in one go! Place all ingredients in the Nutri Ninja and blend.

Did You Know

Avocados are a superfood, worthy of the name. It is one of the healthiest foods you can consume in your diet. They are rich in monounsaturated fats making them a fabulous source of energy when you need to work out. I often have this smoothie a couple of hours before a long training run. In fact it is the very smoothie I drank before I completed a marathon.

Clearer and Younger Looking Skin Smoothies

You can spend all you want on expensive skin creams, if you are not nourishing your body from the inside, it will show on the outside. Eating the right foods will not only be cheaper than the latest skin cream, but you will also reap the benefits across your whole body.

The cells in your skin are constantly shedding and being replaced by younger ones. To support this speedy growth, you need to supply your skin with the right balance of nourishing foods. Fruit and vegetables help to protect the skin from cellular damage due to the powerful abundance of antioxidants that they contain.

Eating a wide range of colourful ingredients will help your skin become more supple, toned, smooth, younger looking and healthy. You will discover that once you are regularly feeding your body with the right foods, your skin will reward you with a blemish and spot free glow.

Essentials for Healthy Skin

Water - Stay hydrated by drinking at least 8 cups of water a day. Your skin needs the moisture and hydration to look fresh and young. Even a little amount of dehydration will dry out your skin and make you look tired.

Essential Fatty Acids - Found in nuts, seeds, avocados and fish. All these will help you skin to stay supple by acting as a natural moisturiser. With their high levels of vitamin E your skin will have a lovely supple look.

Omega 3 and Omega 6 - These cannot be made in your body so need to be taken from your diet. They can be found in oily fish as well as flaxseed, linseeds and walnuts.

Selenium - this powerful antioxidant, which can be found in tomatoes, Brazil Nuts, eggs and broccoli, are great for protecting against sun damage and age spots.

Protect your skin in the sun from harmful rays

Start your day with a glass of water with fresh lemon juice squeezed in it. Lemons contain a lot of vitamin C (as well as other antioxidants) which help reduce blemishes and wrinkles. Lemons are a great detoxifier, helping your body become cleaner on the inside, resulting in healthy and clear skin on the outside.

Blueberry Blast

1 bunch of parsley
1 handful of spinach
1/4 pineapple
2 handfuls of frozen blueberries
250ml of oatmilk
Ice cubes

Making It

Place all of the ingredients in the Nutri Ninja blender. Feel free to substitute the oat milk for an unsweetened nut milk or other healthy liquid alternative.

Did You Know

Eating blueberries can help leave your skin with a softer and younger look and feel. The antioxidants and phytochemicals found in blueberries help to neutralize free radicals which can damage skin cells. Due to the nutrients found in blueberries, they can assist with slowing down the aging process.

Parsley is very rich in calcium, iron and is a complete protein. Parsley is great for rejuvenating and detoxifying the body. It does have a distinctive taste and combines well with spinach. Studies show that parsley can help slow the aging process. Parsley is easy to grow at home too, how about that, really fresh parsley to pick as and when you need it.

Oat milk is high in natural fibre and iron and low in fat. Oats are also said to have properties within them that help with clearer skin by improving the health of it.

Clearer Cucumber

1 handful of spinach
1/2 cucumber
1 kiwi
250ml of coconut water
1 banana
Ice cubes

Making It

Peel the kiwi. Place all the ingredients in your Nutri Ninja and blend.

Did You Know

The skin of a cucumber contains the mineral silicia. Silica can be great for the complexion so is brilliant for people suffering with skin conditions. It also adds elasticity to your skin, great for creating younger looking skin, hooray for the cucumber!

Kiwis are high in vitamin E, an antioxidant known to protect skin from aging too quickly.

Brazilian Beauty

1 handful of spinach
1 banana1 handful of fresh or frozen mango3 brazil nuts1 tbsp ground flax seeds250ml of coconut water or plain water

Making It

Put all the ingredients in the Nutri Ninja cup and blend. The brazil nuts add a lovely creamy taste to the smoothie. Drink and pretend you're on the beaches of Rio.

Did You Know

Brazil nuts are packed full of nutrients. They have an abundance of vitamins, antioxidants and minerals. One important antioxidant mineral that the brazil nut has a lot of is selenium. Selenium helps maintain the elasticity and firmness of your skin. It can also help reduce sun damage.

Mango Tango

1 apple
1 banana
1 handful of fresh or frozen mango
250ml of coconut water or plain water
Ice cubes

Making It

Chop up the apple and banana. Add all the ingredients to the Nutri Ninja blender. Blend the ingredients. Add more liquid if you prefer a thinner consistency.

Did You Know

Mango contains vitamins B6, C and E, all of which help boost your skin. As mangoes are rich in beta-carotene it can help with acne and lack lustre looking skin. Mango can of course also be used externally to help cleanse your skin. Personally, I rather eat it though!

Strawberry Sip

1 handful of spinach
1 handful of romaine lettuce
2 handfuls of fresh or frozen strawberries
1 tbsp of ground flaxseeds
250ml of water
Ice cubes

Making It

Add all the ingredients to the Nutri Ninja and blend.

Did You Know

Ground flaxseeds are plentiful in essential fatty acids which are brilliant for keeping your skin hydrated, soft and smooth looking. It is said that flax seeds may help reduce skin irritations and rashes.

Up the Apples & Pears

1 handfuls of spinach
1 handful of fresh or frozen blueberries
1 apple
1 pear
1 tbsp of ground flaxseeds
250ml of coconut water
Ice cubes

Making It

Add all the ingredients to the Nutri Ninja blender and top up with water if required. Blend for around 30 seconds or until smooth.

Did You Know

Apples are great for cleaning the colon and getting your skin looking clear. They are full of vitamin C which is fantastic for your skin complexion. Apples also contain vitamin Bs which are good for skin problems.

Pears are an anti-aging fruit that can really boost your skin's appearance and health. Pears contain a lot of fibre which is great for your skin. It helps to keep your complexion looking smooth.

Oooh Peachy

1 handful of kale
2 peaches
2 handfuls of grapes
250ml coconut water
Ice cubes

Making It

Place all the ingredients in your Nutri Ninja blender. Blend for approximately 30 seconds. Add more liquid if required.

Did You Know

Peaches contain vitamin C which is a major health benefit for the skin.

Grapes are a great source of flavonoids. Flavonoids are very powerful antioxidants that can help slow down aging. They have a high nutrient content which is important for a healthy body.

Cashew Crunch

1 handful of mixed greens
1/4 pineapple
1 handful of fresh or frozen strawberries
1 handful of cashew nuts
Water
Ice cubes

Making It

Remove the skin from the pineapple and chop. Place all the ingredients in the blender cup and blend for around 30 seconds.

Did You Know

Cashew nuts are rich in selenium and zinc. Selenium works alongside vitamin E which helps to hydrate the skin and reduce skin inflammation. Zinc is great for the immune system and cell growth, helping to renew skin that may have been damaged previously.

Superfood Smoothies

There is no legal or medical definition of what makes a food make it as a super food. In general though, they are foods that are found in nature and rich in nutrients. They are said to have certain health benefits which can help to combat certain ailments and reduce your risk of getting others.

The Green Machine

1 handful of spinach
1 handful of kale
1/2 avocado
1/4 cucumber
Juice of 1 lime
250ml of coconut water
Ice cubes

Making It

Scoop out the flesh of the avocado. Squeeze the juice from 1 lime. Add all the other ingredients. Add more water if required. Blend for 30 seconds or until smooth.
I love this smoothie. The combination of all the green goodness makes me feel like my body is really getting all the nutrients I need. Individually they are all ingredients I wouldn't really eat, but combined in a smoothie like this I love them.

Purple Punch

1 handful of romaine lettuce
250ml frozen mixed berries
1/2 tsp cinnamon
125ml pomegranate juice
50ml of probiotic vanilla yoghurt
Water

Making It

Place all the ingredients in the blender. Blend for 30 seconds. Add water if you want a thinner consistency.

Did You Know

The pomegranate and in particular, pomegranate juice, has remarkable levels of antioxidant properties. Pomegranates are abundantly rich in potassium, fibre, vitamin C, niacin and disease fighting antioxidants.

Top Tip

You could pour the juice into ice cube trays and freeze. The perfect way to get your smoothie super cold and tasty whilst including a superfood.
Cinnamon equals Christmas memories for me, so a welcome addition to any smoothie. Memories aside, cinnamon helps to balance blood sugar levels.

Blueberry Beauties

1 handful of kale
1/2 banana
2 handful of fresh or frozen blueberries
250ml unsweetened almond milk
Ice cubes

Making It

Add all of the ingredients to the Nutri Ninja Blender. If you don't like almond milk feel free to substitute it for coconut water or just plain water. Blend for 30 seconds.

Did You Know

Blueberries are a popular superfood. They are high in numerous vitamins and minerals. They help slow down the signs of ageing. They contain high levels of antioxidants which are said to help protect against many health issues, including heart disease, stroke and gum disease amongst others. They are also reported as helping to enhance eyesight.

Kale Crunch

2 handfuls of kale
1/2 pineapple
1/2 banana
250ml coconut water
Ice cubes

Making It

Place all the ingredients in the Nutri Ninja and blend. Add more coconut water or plain water if required. Blend for around 30 seconds or until smooth.

Did You Know

Kale contains all the essential amino acids and 9 non essential ones. It has an exceptionally high level of protein in it and is a powerful antioxidant.

Oat-tastic

1 pear
1 apple
30g oatmeal
1 tbsp honey
250ml of unsweetened almond milk
Ice cubes

Making It

Chop the apple and pear up, removing the core, leaving the skin on. Add the other ingredients and top up with water if required. Blend for about 30 seconds until smooth.

Did You Know

Oats are a traditional remedy for helping with digestive problems. They are highly nutritious being a good source of protein and high in calcium, potassium and magnesium. They provide us with sustainable energy and make for a fantastic filling addition to any smoothie.

Hey Honey

1 handful of romaine lettuce
1 handful of watercress
1 tbsp of honey
1 handful of fresh or frozen blueberries
1 tbsp of chia seeds
250ml of coconut water
Ice cubes

Making It

Add all of the ingredients to your Nutri Ninja. Add more water if required. Blend for around 30 seconds or until smooth.

Did You Know

Winnie Pooh was on to something with his love of honey. Honey is a powerful addition to your daily diet. This isn't a new finding - the health benefits of honey go back to early Greek, Roman, Vedic and Islamic texts. The list of healing properties and benefits of honey is a book all in itself, there are countless reports and studies to show that honey is a powerhouse of nutrients that can help soothe coughs, boost memory, help with allergies and plenty more.

Watercress is great for vitamin deficiencies and makes a tasty addition to any smoothie. When eaten raw, watercress is a rich source of minerals and vitamins. It contains an abundance of vitamin K and vitamin A which are great for your bones and eye well-being. Watercress also has high levels of antioxidants.

Go Nuts

1 handful of spinach
1 handful of mixed nuts (try a variety but definitely include walnuts)
1/2 banana
250ml of coconut water
Ice cubes

Making It

Add all the ingredients. Top up with water if required. Blend for around 30 seconds or until smooth.

Did You Know

Walnuts are a rich source of omega-3 fatty acids. They are also a good source of fibre and protein. Walnuts are the golden star of nuts with the highest overall antioxidant activity of them all.

The Blackberry

1 stick of celery
1 handful of fresh or frozen blackberries
2 kiwis
Half a lemon (unwaxed)
250ml coconut water

Making It

Chop the ingredients and place them all in the blender. Blend for 30 seconds.

Did You Know

Blackberries have a high concentration of antioxidants. They are low in calories, high in fibre and rich in nutrients. They have a lot of fibre and are almost fat free, making them a perfect addition for a healthy smoothie. Blackberries has folic acid and vitamins C and K, all which are great for your joints and bones. Plus they taste great!

Easy Squeezy

1 handful of spinach
2 apples
1/2 lemon (unwaxed)
Water
Ice Cubes

Making It

Chop apples. If you are not using an unwaxed lemon make sure you peel it. Add all ingredients and top up with the desired amount of water. Blend for around 30 seconds or until smooth.

Did You Know

Studies have shown that eating an apple a day can lower bad cholesterol in the blood. Apples contain polyphenol antioxidants which are said to lower blood oxidation.

Lemon juice is a great alkalizer for the body. Did you know when we have too much acid in our body our energy levels drop and our immune systems do not work at their full ability? Lemon is said to be great at detoxing your body.

A great drink that I have grown to love is hot water with the juice of half a lemon. It is meant to improve liver function and help eliminate kidney stones.

Healthy Heart Smoothies

Getting regular exercise combined with eating nutrient rich healthy food is something your heart will love you for. And a happy heart is a healthy heart. Eating a well balanced diet rich in fruits and vegetables will ensure that your risk of developing heart disease is significantly reduced. The more nutrients and healthy fats that you consume, the better. Drinking a smoothie a day will go a long way to making this possible. You can make sure that your heart is getting all the fibre it needs whilst ensuring your cholesterol stays low.

Flaxseed, oatmeal, walnuts, soy milk, blueberries, carrots, spinach, broccoli, dark chocolate (lowers blood pressure).

Heart Beet

1 handful of kale
1/2 beetroot
1 apple
1 carrot
1/2 lemon (unwaxed)
1 table spoon of ground flaxseed
Water
Ice cubes

Making It

As mentioned elsewhere in this book, beetroot can have a powerful taste. If you find it too strong please feel free to juice the beetroot or use a lower quantity. Add all the ingredients into the Nutri Ninja cup. Top up with water. Blend for around 30 seconds or until smooth.

Did You Know

Beetroot is a powerful blood cleanser and tonic. Beetroot promotes a healthy digestive system as well as a healthy heart. Beetroot is a great blood builder and fortifier.

Avocado Baby

1 handful of mixed greens
1/2 ripe avocado
1/2 banana
1 handful of fresh or frozen strawberries
Water
Ice cubes

Making It

Scoop out the flesh of the avocado. Add all the ingredients to the Nutri Ninja blender cup. Top up with water or other liquid. Blend for around 30 seconds.

Did You Know

Avocados can aid in lowering our risk of heart disease due to their monounsaturated fatty acid content. The vitamin B-6 and folic acid also plays a part in supporting a healthy heart.

I Heart Chocolate

1 handful of spinach
1 handful of frozen raspberries
1 banana
2 squares of grated dark chocolate (minimum 75% cocoa content)
1 table spoon of peanut butter (natural if possible)
250ml of coconut water
Ice cubes

Making It

Grate the chocolate. Place all the ingredients in the blender cup and blend for about 30 seconds. Add more liquid if you require a thinner drink.

Did You Know

Studies show that dark chocolate can help lower your blood pressure. By eating good quality dark chocolate a few times a week you can help prevent the formation of blood clots along with improve the blood flow to your heart.

Peanut butter (if of the natural variety) has around 75% unsaturated fats which helps keep your heart healthy. The protein and fat in natural peanut butter will keep you feeling fuller for longer.

Acai Heart

1 handful of mixed greens
1 tbsp of acai berries (fresh, dried or powdered)
1 handful of fresh or frozen blueberries
250ml of soy milk/unsweetened nut milk
Ice cubes

Making It

Add all the ingredients to the Nutri Ninja cup and blend. Top up with water if required. Acai berries can be purchased from some supermarkets and all health food stores.

Did You Know

Commonly found in the rain forests of the Amazon, acai berries are very high in antioxidants. They are said to help prevent blood clots by improving overall blood circulation and relaxing the blood vessels.

Heart Healthy Super Greens

1 handful of spinach
1 handful of kale
1 apple
1 carrot
1 tbsp of mixed seeds
250ml of coconut Water
Ice cubes

Making It

Add all the ingredients to the blender. Feel free to add more seeds if you wish. Top up with water if required. Blend for around 30 seconds.

Did You Know

You will probably have seen spinach and kale feature quite heavily throughout this book, and with good reason. They are both so incredibly good for you, with so many health benefits. Kale can help lower cholesterol levels. Kale is low in calories, high in fibre and has zero fat. Spinach has high levels of potassium and low levels of sodium, the composition of these minerals helps to lower blood pressure.

Smoothie Remedies

It is always worth looking at your diet when you start suffering from some common ailments. If our bodies are lacking in nutrients we can help ourselves by consuming the right foods.

By making a few simple lifestyle changes and implementing particular foods into our diet we can help protect and promote vibrant health.

Eating raw foods when combined with exercise, rest and the right attitude can go a long way to making you feel better and less reliant on quick fixes.

(If you are taking medication please remember to consult a doctor before making any decisions about stopping them.)

The Anti-Sneeze

1 apple
1/2 pineapple
1cm ginger
1/2 lemon (unwaxed)
1 tbsp of honey
Water
Ice cubes

Making It

Peel the pineapple and chop. Peel the skin from the lemon if you are using the unwaxed variety. Add all ingredients to the blender. Top up with water. Blend for around 30 seconds.

Did You Know

If you suffer from hay fever you will know the frustrations of sneezing and feeling blocked up, amongst other ailments. Consuming the combination of these ingredients may go some way to giving you some relief. Pineapple contains bromeline which is an enzyme that can aid in dissolving excess mucus. Ginger is a natural decongestant and honey has been said to help fight off the symptoms of hayfever, especially if you are using a locally produced honey.

Abundantly Rich Smoothie

1 handful of spinach
1 handful of kale
1 handful of fresh or frozen blueberries
1 apple
1 tbsp ground flaxseeds
1 tbsp of honey
Water
Ice cubes

Making It

Add all the ingredients to the Nutri Ninja blender. Top up with water. Blend for around 30 seconds.

Did You Know

You can add a tablespoon of ground flaxseeds to any smoothie (but don't have more than 2 tablespoons in a day as the husks contain compounds that can be toxic in high doses.) The amazing health giving properties of flaxseed are recognized around the world. They are a rich source of dietary fibre which can help relieve constipation. Other benefits include essential fatty acids, in particular omega 3 and omega 6.

Cause I Eats Me Spinach

2 handfuls of spinach
1 carrot
3 ready to eat dried apricots
1/2 lemon (unwaxed)
250ml coconut water
Ice cubes

Making It

Place all the ingredients in the Nutri Ninja blender. Add more water or liquid if required.

Did You Know

Popeye had the right idea. Spinach is one of the healthiest foods you can eat. Spinach is one of the best sources of folate which is necessary for brain and cardiovascular health. If you suffer from anaemia as a result of low iron levels, spinach is a fantastic remedy, containing nearly twice as much iron as most other greens.

Dried apricots are another great source of iron, meaning the combination of these two iron rich foods in one smoothie will do wonders for your iron, and in turn, energy levels.

Going Back to Your Roots

1 handful of romaine lettuce
1/2 raw beetroot
1 carrot
1cm of ginger
1/2 lemon (unwaxed)
Water
Ice cubes

Making It

Add all the ingredients to the Nutri Ninja. If you don't like the strong taste of raw beetroot you may want to juice it instead. Add more water or liquid if required.

Did You Know

Beetroot has many amazing health benefits. It is great for cleansing the liver, increasing iron levels and helping lower blood pressure.

Winter Booster

1 apple
Juice from 2 oranges
2 passion fruits
1 handful of fresh or frozen mango
Half a lemon (unwaxed)
1 tsp of echinacea powder
Water
Ice cubes

Making It

Chop the apple. You can add the whole oranges (peeled) if you prefer. Scoop out the pulp of the passion fruits. Add all ingredients to the Nutri Ninja and top up with water. Blend for around 30 seconds. Echinacea can be bought from any health store or ordered online. Passion fruits are best when they are ripe.

Did You Know

This is the perfect smoothie to fight off cold and flu. Echinacea, mango, pineapple and oranges are all rich in vitamin C

The Pick Me Up

1 handful of spinach
1 apple
1 orange
1 tbsp honey
1cm of fresh root ginger
1 handful of fresh or frozen mango
1/4 pineapple
250ml of coconut water
Ice cubes

Making It

There is quite a lot to squeeze into this smoothie. I made this recently for my son when he was feeling run down after a bout of a winter cold virus. He loved the taste of it and it really did perk him up. Chop the apple, peel the orange (if you don't like bits, juice it instead.) Peel the pineapple and chop it up. Blend everything together.

Did You Know

When you are feeling run down a smoothie is a quick way to get a lot of vitamins and nutrients into your system. All of these ingredients are great for boosting your immune system due to the amount of vitamin C present. The pineapple can help dissolve excess mucus so particularly good when you have a cold.

Prune Relief

2 handfuls of kale
1 banana
1 pear
3 dried prunes (pitted)
250ml water
Ice cubes

Making It

Place all the ingredients in the blender. You may want to blend for a bit longer than the 30 seconds if the prunes haven't quite got to a smooth enough consistency.

Did You Know

Prunes are the most natural laxative you can get. If you struggle with constipation then the combination of the prunes with the soluble fibre of the apples and pears, will have you relieved soon enough. Prunes are also a brilliant source of beta carotene and vitamin K.

Ginger Zest

2 carrots
1 handful of fresh or frozen mango
1/4 cucumber
1cm ginger
1/2 lemon (unwaxed)
Water
Ice cubes

Making It

Add all the ingredients to the Nutri Ninja. If you are not using unwaxed lemons, peel the skin off and just add the flesh. Top up with water. Blend for around 30 seconds.

Did You Know

Fresh root ginger is a fantastic natural cure for unsettled stomachs and indigestion. It is a natural antibiotic and decongestant. Ginger is also warming and soothing and a favourite natural remedy for colds.

Breakfast Smoothies

It's been said many times before, breakfast is the most important meal of the day. If I ever skip breakfast I start to feel *really* hungry by 10am. This is when I'm at my weakest, when I'm really hungry, and I find myself reaching for a quick fix, often unhealthy, energy boost.

By incorporating a smoothie into your breakfast routine, you will be setting yourself up for a healthy and productive day, filling your body up with nature's finest fuel. Make extra so that you can sip on some mid morning.

Sometimes I will just have a smoothie for breakfast, depending on how I am feeling and what I am doing. I quite often go for a run in the morning, so it makes sense for me to just have a smoothie. I find it helpful to plan the night before what smoothie I am going to have, that way I have no excuse to skip it when I am in a rush in the morning.

Rocket Boost

1 handful of fresh or frozen raspberries
1 handful of fresh or frozen blueberries
200ml oat milk
3 tablespoons of live natural yoghurt
1 tablespoon of honey

Making It

Place all of the ingredients in the Nutri Ninja cup and blend for 30 seconds. Top up with water or more oat milk if required. If you don't like yoghurt then feel free to add less or leave it out altogether.

Did You Know

Oat milk is made with presoaked oat groats (hulled grains broken down.) Oat milk has a slightly sweet but mild taste. It makes for a great substitute for milk. It is very low in fat and is lactose free. It makes for a great vegan alternative. Oatmilk contains 15 vitamins and 10 minerals. It has more vitamin A than cow's milk. It is also high in iron so great for any anemia sufferers out there.

Berry Tasty

1 large apple
1 handful of fresh or frozen raspberries
1 handful of fresh or frozen strawberries
1 orange (or the juice of one)
250ml coconut water
Ice cubes

Making It

Chop up the apple, removing the core. Add all the ingredients to the Nutri Ninja blender. Top up with more water if required. Blend for 30 seconds or until smooth.

Did You Know

Berries make a brilliant start to the day and feel like quite a treat. They are a great way of getting antioxidants and phytonutrients into your system. They are great for your immune system and disease fighting abilities. Don't underestimate the power of the berries.

Filling Breakfast Smoothie

1 pear
1 banana
50g muesli
1 tbsp natural maple syrup
200ml unsweetened soy milk

Making It

Chop the pear and add all the ingredients to your Nutri Ninja. Top up with water if required. Blend for 30 seconds or until smooth.

Did You Know

Maple Syrup can boost your immune system, sooth your stomach and help ageing skin. When you buy maple syrup make sure that 'maple syrup' is the only ingredient listed. It is loaded with antioxidants in the form of polyphenols. Maple syrup also contains essential nutrients like zinc and manganese. Zinc is great for resisting illness and manganese helps protect immune cells from damage.

Kicking K

3 kiwis
2 stick celery
1 banana
Water
Ice Cubes

Making It

Place all ingredients in the cup, fill with water up to the max line. If you prefer a thicker smoothie substitute the water for unsweetened almond milk, oat milk, or another healthy liquid alternative.

Did You Know

Kiwis are a very nutrient rich fruit containing vitamins C, E and beta-carotene. They are full of healthy minerals including calcium, magnesium, phosphorus, potassium and sodium. They are great for providing you with an energy boost to start the day. The high vitamin C content will help strengthen your immune system too.

Great Greens

1 handful of spinach
1 handful of kale
1/4 cucumber
1/4 medium pineapple
1/2 ripe avocado
250ml coconut water
Ice cubes

Making It

Scoop out the flesh from a ripe avocado. Place all ingredients in the Nutri Ninja and blend. Add more liquid if required.

Did You Know

Avocados are a great way to set you up for a healthy day. They contain all the vital vitamins, minerals and fats required to keep you in peak condition. They are filling (in a good way) so will keep you feeling fuller for longer.

Smoothies for Kids

It feels really great to know that not only myself, but the children too, are getting their full recommendation of vitamins and nutrients, in the healthiest style, before they've even left for school in the morning. Not only that, they are enjoying it too. Don't get me wrong, we are not replacing the children's meals with smoothies. We still serve up an array of vegetables with their evening meals, but if there is the odd day they don't feel like eating them, I don't feel like I need to do battle with them to eat those last few peas they've cunningly hidden under their spoon. I know that they have already fuelled their bodies with nutrients from the best possible sources. The extras at mealtimes are the icing on the cake, so to speak.

These smoothies are not exclusively for the kiddies though. You'll reap the rewards of drinking them too. Allow your children to be really involved in the process - from choosing the recipe, picking up the ingredients and then making the smoothie. Discuss with them what nutrients are in each smoothie and what brilliance they are doing for their bodies. It sets them up for fantastic healthy habits for both now and adulthood.

Don't forget you can turn many of these smoothies into yummy and nutritious ice lollies.

Captain Bright Eye

3 medium carrots
1cm of ginger
Juice from 2 oranges
250ml of coconut water (or plain water)
Ice cubes

Making It

Add all the ingredients to the Nutri Ninja Blender. You may want to start with small amounts of ginger if your child isn't used to the taste. Just grate a little bit in and build up according to taste.

Did You Know

Carrots are naturally sweet, making them an excellent vegetable to include in a kid's smoothie. They are high in fibre and carotenoids. But can they really make you see in the dark? Or was that just a ploy to get us, as children ourselves, to eat up all our carrots? Well, actually, there is some truth in it. They contain a lot of Vitamin A which helps you to produce rhodopsin. Rhodopsin is a purple pigment that your eyes need in order to see in dim light. So although you won't have quite the superpowers of night vision that you were led to believe, you will be able to see in some lights.

Strawberry Surprise

1 handful of spinach
2 handfuls of fresh or frozen strawberries
1 orange
Water
Ice cubes

Making It

Peel the orange and put segments into the blender. Add all the other ingredients and fill the water up to the max line. If you or your little one isn't keen on 'bits' then feel free to squeeze the juice out of the orange instead of putting the whole fruit in.

Did You Know

Strawberries are a fantastic source of vitamin C. Weight for weight they have more vitamin C than an orange. The seeds in strawberries provide fibre which helps with constipation.

Gone Bananas

1 handful of kale
1 handful of fresh or frozen strawberries
1 banana
250ml of coconut water (or other liquid to thin)
Ice cubes

Making It

Place all the ingredients in the Nutri Ninja and blend. Add more banana or strawberries if you prefer a thicker smoothie.

Did You Know

Bananas are great for an energy pick me up (as if the little monkeys ever require more energy!) and can make you feel less tired. Bananas are very high in potassium, an electrolyte that is vital for your body's function. Potassium helps to build proteins and maintain normal body growth. Bananas mixed with strawberries make a delicious combination.

Fruitylicious

Juice from 2 oranges
2 kiwis
1 Pear
Water
Ice cubes

Making It

Juice 2 orange, or if you don't mind bits just put the whole orange in the blender (without the skin.) Peel and cut the kiwis. Chop the pear up but leave the skin on. Add all the ingredients. Top up with water. Blend for about 30 seconds.

Peany B Booster

1 handful of spinach
1 tablespoon of peanut butter (natural if possible)
1 ripe banana
250ml unsweetened soy milk or an alternative recommended liquid.
Ice cubes

Making It

Place all of the ingredients in the Nutri Ninja and blend. If you can use a natural type of peanut butter even better. The regular peanut butter tends to have additives, preservatives, added sugar and salt.

Did You Know

Peanut butter is a staple in our household. Natural peanut butter should just have peanuts and salt listed as the ingredients. Peanut butter has potassium and protein in it together with fibre, healthy fats, vitamin E, antioxidants and plenty of magnesium to make your bones and muscles strong.

Mango Mayhem

1 handful of fresh or frozen mango
1/4 pineapple
1 apple
1/2 cucumber
250ml of coconut water (or water)
Ice cubes

Making It

Remove the skin from the pineapple and chop. Place all the ingredients into the blender. Add more water or liquid if you require a thinner consistency.

Did You Know

Mango is great for stimulating the immune system. It is a fantastic source of vitamins C and A as well as potassium. Kids love the taste of mango, it creates a deliciously smooth and tasty smoothie.

Super Green Machine

1 handful of spinach
1 handful of romaine lettuce
1 apple
1/2 ripe avocado
Half lime
1 tsp of honey
Water
Ice cubes

Making It

Chop the apple up. Scoop the avocado out of the skin. Add all the ingredients into the Nutri Ninja and fill with water to the max line. Blend for 30 seconds. Add more water if you prefer a thinner drink.

Did You Know

Avocado is perfect for ensuring your child is getting a balanced and nutritious diet. They are packed full of a 6 requirements for a healthy body: fat, protein, water, natural sugar, minerals and vitamins. Avocados are a great source of essential natural fats, the kind children need daily in their diet.

The Chocolate Monster

1 banana
2 squares of 75% cocoa content chocolate, grated
1 handful of frozen or fresh strawberries
250ml of coconut water
Ice cubes

Making It

Grate the chocolate. Place all the ingredients in the blender. Add more water if required. Add another banana or maybe even a scoop of yoghurt or vanilla ice cream to turn this into a tasty dessert.

The Secret Super Booster

2 broccoli florets
1 apple
1 carrot
1 handful of frozen strawberries
250ml of water

Making It

Put all ingredients in blender. Add more water if needed.

Did You Know

We keep on telling them how good broccoli is. If they don't believe you maybe a few of these smoothies will change their minds. Broccoli is a really important ingredient for a healthy diet. Broccoli has oodles of antibacterial and antiviral nutrients. It also has almost as much calcium as milk. Perfect for growing children. What's more, broccoli has almost twice as much protein as steak - who'd have thought it?

Peachy Lemonade

1 apple
2 peaches
Juice of half a lemon
100ml of coconut water
150ml of carbonated water (or you may know it as sparkling water)
Ice cubes

Making It

Place all the ingredients in the Nutri Ninja apart from the carbonated water. Blend. Add carbonated water to turn this delicious drink into lemonade, but not as they know it.

Did You Know

Peaches are a rich source of beta carotene which can be great vision health. Peaches have a wide range of vitamins and minerals. Peaches are also fibrous which is great for digestion and preventing constipation.

SOUP RECIPE BOOK

Using a Nutri Ninja

Since we bought our Nutri Ninja last year, it has been heavily in use every single day. It really has become a very versatile and dependable appliance in our kitchen. We used to just make smoothies with it, but as we love soup, we decided to start experimenting with making that in the blender too. The results have been fantastic, and we are testing out new recipes all the time. I love the simplicity of putting everything in a saucepan to cook and then blending it on high speed in the Nutri Ninja.

Aside from the delicious taste of homemade soup, the recipes also offer a huge amount of nutritional health benefits. I have tried to list as many of those benefits where I can under each recipe.

Which Blender?

The recipes in this book are aimed at all high power blenders. We personally use the Nutri Ninja BL450, but they can also be used in the Nutri Ninja Professional IQ BL480, the popular Nutribullet or any high powered blender.

Using the Nutri Ninja Blender for Soup

Follow the recipe instructions and allow the contents to cool to room temperature before pouring into the Nutri Ninja cup. This is as per the manufacturer's instructions in order to prevent any accidents with boiling contents and to protect your appliance from damage. I might not always wait until it is completely room temperature but that is my own choice. Always follow the manufacturer's guidelines and don't fill the cups above the 'max' line.

As a guideline, blend for about 30 seconds. Some recipes, depending on the ingredients, may require a little longer to be completely smooth.

Equipment

You shouldn't really need much more than what is already in your kitchen.

a medium to large size saucepan

a measuring jug

a frying pan

a garlic crusher

a grater

Preparing the Ingredients

The recipes are all very simple and fuss free to prepare. The ingredients are all easy to source from your local shops, or if you are fortunate enough, straight from your vegetable patch.

Many of the recipes include onion and garlic - this is intentional! They add the perfect aromatic taste to soups, not to mention the health benefits they provide. However, if you are not a fan, please feel free to reduce the amount or leave out. Onions and garlic are part of the allium family of vegetables, along with leeks. They are great for strengthening your immune system and combatting infection. Onions are also rich in flavonoids which can help protect you from heart disease. Crushing or chopping garlic prior to cooking, and leaving for 5 to 10 minutes, helps to retain the healthy benefits.

All of the recipes have some kind of stock included, either vegetable or chicken stock. You can choose whether you want to make the stock yourself (please see page 75 for some stock recipes) or buy shop made stock. There is something satisfying about making everything from scratch, but sometimes the reality is we don't always have the time. There is a huge choice these days for premade stock so just go with what suits you best.

Feel free to add more or less liquid stock when cooking your soup, according to how thick or thin you like it. You can also use hot water to thin the soup out.

The Quantities

All of these recipes are designed to be made in the larger of the cups (650ml). However, the exact amount you get is always subjective; not all vegetable sizes are created equal! You may not be able to fit it all in (don't go over the max line), if this is the case, just blend it in two separate batches.

Whether the finished soup provides enough for 1 or 2 servings is again subjective. If I am having one of the recipes as my lunch with some bread on the side, I might have the whole lot. However, if it is an afternoon snack (yes I do have them as snacks to perk me up sometimes!) or as a starter, I will probably only have half of it.

The soup can be stored in a sealed container in the fridge for a few days, or frozen for up to 3 months.

Vegetable Soup

Ingredients

1 small red onion, chopped
1 medium carrot, chopped
1 parsnip, chopped
1 sweet potato, chopped
1 leek, chopped
Half of 1 red chilli, seeded and finely chopped (adjust quantity of chilli depending on how hot you like it!)
350ml vegetable stock
1 tablespoon of olive oil

Making It

1. Heat the olive oil in a large saucepan
2. Add the vegetables (onion, carrots, parsnip, leek, sweet potato) and cook for about 5 minutes
3. Add the water and bring to the boil. Cover and cook for a further 20 minutes
4. Allow to cool to room temperature.
5. Pour contents of saucepan into your blender and blend for about 30 seconds until completely smooth. Add more stock or hot water if required.
6. Pour contents back in to the saucepan and add the chilli. Alter the consistency with a little stock or hot water if desired. Season with salt and pepper if required.
7. Simmer for 10 minutes and serve.

Health Benefits

Chillis not only taste good, they also speed up your metabolism. They raise your endorphin levels making you feel better.

Carrots are naturally sweet and high in fibre and carotenoids. The high fibre content is great for weight management, making you feel fuller for longer.

Sweet Potatoes are high in beta-carotene, vitamin A and vitamin C. The vitamin A can help support healthy blood cell development.

Leeks are part of the onion and garlic family and offer a great array of health benefits. Leeks are high in the antioxidant polyphenol and the flavonoid kaempferol, which play a part in protecting our blood vessels and cells from damage. The allicin found in leeks can help fight dangerous free radicals in your body. Leeks are also low in calories yet help to make you feel full. Leeks also contain high levels of vitamin K and A.

Carrot and Ginger

Ingredients

1 tbsp. of olive oil
4 medium carrots, chopped
2 teaspoon of grated ginger
1 small onion, chopped
350ml of chicken stock

Making It

1. Heat the olive oil in a medium saucepan and add the onions. Cook on a gentle heat for 5 minutes. Do not allow to go brown.
2. Add the chopped carrots, grated ginger and chicken stock. Bring to the boil and then cover and simmer for about 15-20 minutes, or until the carrots are soft.
3. Allow to cool to room temperature.
4. Pour contents in to your Nutri Ninja and blend for about 30 seconds or until smooth. Add more stock or hot water if required.
5. Return contents to the saucepan and season if required.
6. Heat gently and serve.

Health Benefits

Not only does fresh rootginger add a lovely warming zing to a soup dish, ginger is also well known for its incredible health benefits. It is full of nutrients that are very beneficial for your body and brain.

It is also particularly great for unsettled stomachs. Ginger is a known natural remedy for colds and flu, with powerful antioxidant and anti-inflammatory benefits.

Butternut Squash

Ingredients

20g of butter
1 medium potato (Maris Piper are best but any will do)
1 butternut squash with seeds removed
300ml of vegetable stock
40ml of single cream (optional)

Making It

1. Place the halved and deseeded butternut squash in a suitably sized roasting tin. Place the butter around the squash.
2. Bake in a preheated oven (gas mark 3 or 160 C) for about 1 hour
3. Cook the potatoes and vegetable stock in a saucepan until the potatoes are soft (about 20 minutes.)
4. Once the butternut squash is cooked and softened scoop out the flesh (make sure it isn't too hot).
5. Allow to cool to room temperature.
6. Add both the potatoes and the scooped out squash to the Nutri Ninja. Blend for about 30 seconds or until smooth. Add more stock or hot water if required.
7. Pour the contents into a saucepan and add the single cream.
8. Season with salt and pepper if required.
9. Reheat on a low heat and serve.

Health Benefits

Butternut squash is both low in fat and high in dietary fibre, so not only does it make you feel fuller for longer, it is also a good choice for your heart. Butternut squash is high in vitamin B6, essential for both your immune system and nervous system. It also contains high levels of potassium which is vital for healthy bones.

Leek and Potato

Ingredients

1 medium onion, chopped
1 leek, finely chopped
1 tbsp. olive oil
1 medium potato (Maris Piper if possible)
350ml of vegetable stock
40ml of single cream (optional)
40ml of milk

Making It

1. Heat the oil in a medium saucepan and add the chopped onion and 1/2 of the finely chopped leek. Cook gently for about 10 minutes until the onion is soft.
2. Chop up the potatoes and add to the saucepan. Cook for a further 3 minutes, stirring continuously.
3. Add the water and bring to the boil. Cover the saucepan and simmer for about 10 minutes (or until the potatoes and leek are soft).
4. Allow the contents to cool to room temperature.
5. Pour the contents into the Nutri Ninja and blend for about 30 seconds or until smooth. Add more stock or hot water if required.
6. Pour back into the saucepan and add the remaining chopped leek. Cook on a gentle heat for about 10 minutes, stirring often.
7. Add in the cream and milk and stir whilst reheating gently.
8. Season with salt and pepper if required. Serve.

Health Benefits

Leeks are part of the onion and garlic family and offer a great array of health benefits. Leeks are high in the antioxidant polyphenol and the flavonoid kaempferol, which play a part in protecting our blood vessels and cells from damage. The allicin found in leeks can help fight dangerous free radicals in your body. Leeks are also low in calories yet help to make you feel full. Leeks also contain high levels of vitamin K and A.

Potatoes support heart health. They are high in fibre and low in cholesterol, rich in potassium, iron, vitamin B-6 and vitamin C. So not only do they taste great, they are also good for our health. The fibre content found in potatoes helps keep us feeling fuller for longer.

Zesty Chicken Soup

Ingredients

1 tbsp. of olive oil
1 cooked chicken breast, shredded
350ml of chicken stock
1 small leek, chopped
1 small potato, chopped (any will do, but I like to use Maris Piper)
2 oranges (as you will be using the skin try and buy organic)
50ml milk
40ml of single cream

Making It

1. Heat the olive oil in a saucepan and add the chopped leeks. Cook gently until soft (about 10 minutes).
2. Add the potato and chicken stock and bring to the boil. Simmer for about 20 minutes.
3. Allow to cool to room temperature.
4. Pour the contents into the Nutri Ninja and blend for about 30 seconds or until smooth. Add more stock or hot water if required.
5. Return the contents to the saucepan and add the shredded chicken. Add the juice and zest of one orange. Peel the other orange and separate the segments out and then chop them into smaller chunks. Add the chopped segments to the soup. Cook on a gentle heat for about 5 minutes.
6. Add the cream and milk and simmer gently for about 5 minutes.
7. Season with salt and pepper if required. Serve.

Health Benefits

Oranges are of course one of the healthiest fruits known to us. The oranges in this recipe add a lovely sweet tang to this soup. The high concentration of vitamin C found within oranges is vital for a healthy immune system. Oranges are full of dietary fibre making them great for your digestive system. The beta-carotene found in oranges help to keep your skin looking young by protecting the cells from damage. Chicken has a high protein content, vital for healthy bones, skin, muscles and blood. It also contains the whole range of vitamin B, great for a healthy metabolism. Chicken is also rich in selenium, a mineral rich in antioxidant properties.

Tomato Soup

Ingredients

1 tbsp. of olive oil
1 medium onion, finely chopped
1 garlic clove, crushed
2 to 3 handfuls of ripe cherry tomatoes, roughly chopped
2 teaspoons of lemon juice
350ml of vegetable stock
25ml milk
50ml of single cream

Making It

1. Heat the oil gently in a saucepan. Add the chopped onions and garlic, cooking gently for about 10 minutes or until soft. Do not allow to brown.
2. Add the tomatoes and cook for a further 10 minutes. Add in the water and lemon juice and simmer for a further 5 minute.
3. Allow to cool to room temperature.
4. Pour the contents into the Nutri Ninja and blend for 30 seconds or until smooth. Add more stock or hot water if required.
5. Return the contents to the saucepan and stir in the cream and milk over a gentle heat.
6. Season with salt and pepper if required. Serve.

Health Benefits

Cherry tomatoes are low in calories and high in nutritious benefits. Cherry tomatoes contain protein, fibre, vitamin C as well as vitamin B-6, a vitamin that helps produce red blood cells and supports brain function. The vitamin A found in the tomatoes help to keep eyes healthy as well as your kidneys, lungs and heart functioning properly.

Cool Avocado Soup

Ingredients

1 large ripe avocado
300ml of coconut milk
2 ice cubes
3 cm of chopped cucumber
1 tbsp. lemon juice
Salt and freshly ground pepper to season, if required

Making It

Make this just before you want to eat it (allowing time to chill in the fridge).
1. Scoop the flesh from the ripe avocado and place in the Nutri Ninja.
2. Add the lemon juice, coconut milk, cucumber and ice cubes. Blend for about 30 seconds until smooth. If the texture is too thick, add a little cold water to thin.
3. If required, season with salt and pepper to taste.
4. Put in the fridge for about an hour to chill. Serve.

Health Benefits

Avocadoes are among the world's healthiest foods. They are high in healthy fats and a great source of fibre. They are high in vitamin E, potassium and iron. The vitamin B-6 and folic acid also play a part in supporting a healthy heart.

Coconut milk is a great alternative to milk, and is also highly nutritious. Coconuts are rich in iron, sodium, selenium, calcium, magnesium, phosphorous, fibre, vitamins B1, B3, B5 B 6 and C & E. Coconut milk is high in saturated fats but it is much healthier than other saturated fat products. Lauric acid is the main saturated fat found in coconut milk, which is said to help promote brain development and bone health. Just check on the carton/tin before buying to make sure there are no added extras to the milk. Even better, why not try making your own?

Garlic Lentil Soup

Ingredients

1 small onion, chopped
1 tbsp. of olive oil
125g of split red lentils
300ml of vegetable stock
1 tbsp. of lemon juice
2 crushed garlic cloves
Salt and freshly ground pepper to taste

Making It

1. Heat the oil in a saucepan. Add the onion and cook for about 5 minutes or until the onion is slightly browned.
2. Add the red lentils and vegetable stock and bring to the boil. Simmer for about 20 minutes. The lentils should turn a golden colour and be soft.
3. Allow to cool to room temperature.
4. Pour the contents of the saucepan into the Nutri Ninja and blend for about 30 seconds or until smooth. If the soup is too thick, add some water to change the consistency.
5. Return the contents to the saucepan and add the lemon juice. If required, season with salt and pepper to taste.
6. Fry the other small chopped onion and 2 crushed garlic gloves in 1 tablespoon of olive oil until softened.
7. Add to the saucepan and reheat over a gentle heat and serve.

Health Benefits

Red lentils, from the legume family, are a great source of protein. They are high in fibre, making you feel fuller for longer. They are fat free and high in a range of nutrients. They have high levels of folic acid, essential for the nervous system and healthy blood cells. Lentils are also a good source of iron, and unlike red meat, do not contain the fat. Iron is vital for maintaining energy levels and is especially important for growing children and menstruating women.

Garlic isn't just for warding off the mosquitoes. Garlic has been used for medicinal purposes for thousands of years. Garlic has a compound in it called Allicin, which is what gives out the distinctively strong garlic smell and taste. Garlic is a good source of vitamin C, selenium, manganese and vitamin B6. Garlic is said to be good for reducing the risk of heart disease and lowering cholesterol levels. Garlic is also a good infection fighter against colds and viruses.

Tomato and Cashew Nut Soup

Ingredients

This is a bit of a spin on the earlier tomato soup recipe but with an extra twist of the cashew nut.

1 tbsp. of olive oil

1 large onion, finely chopped

1 crushed garlic clove

2 to 3 handfuls of ripe cherry tomatoes, roughly chopped

1 tbsp. of lemon juice

350ml of vegetable stock

25ml milk

50ml of single cream

4 cashew nuts

Making It

1. Heat the oil gently in a saucepan. Add the chopped onions and garlic, cooking gently for about 5 minutes or until soft. Do not allow to brown.

2. Add the tomatoes and cook for a further 10 minutes. Add in the vegetable stock and lemon juice and simmer for a further 5 minutes.

3. Allow to cool to room temperature.

4. Pour the contents into the Nutri Ninja, adding the 4 cashew nuts. Blend for 30 seconds or until smooth. Add more stock or hot water if required.

5. Return the contents to the saucepan and stir in the cream and milk over a gentle heat.

6. Season with salt and pepper if required. Serve.

Health Benefits

Cashew nuts add a deliciously succulent flavour to this soup dish, with the added benefit of being really good for you. The cashew nut is packed full with nutrients and high levels of essential minerals including iron, zinc, copper, magnesium, phosphorus and manganese. Cashew nuts are high in healthy fats but contain zero levels of cholesterol. If eaten in moderation, cashew nuts can help with weight loss and weight maintenance. They contain a high level of dietary fibre, making you feel fuller for longer.

Cherry tomatoes are low in calories and high in nutritious benefits. Cherry tomatoes contain protein, fibre, vitamin C as well as vitamin B-6, a vitamin that helps produce red blood cells and supports brain function. The vitamin A found in the tomatoes help to keep eyes healthy as well as your kidneys, lungs and heart functioning properly.

Gazpacho

A classic and simple soup to make, perfect for a warm summers day.

Ingredients

2 tbsp. olive oil
1 medium onion, chopped
1 garlic clove, crushed
1 tin of chopped tomatoes
1 tsp red wine vinegar
Salt and freshly ground pepper to season

Making It

1. Place the tomatoes (still in their juice) with the chopped onion and crushed garlic in the Nutri Ninja. Blend for about 20 seconds. Add a little cold water if you prefer a thinner consistency.
2. Add the red wine vinegar, olive oil and a little salt and pepper. Blend for a further 10 seconds.
3. Put in the fridge to chill (about an hour should do).
4. If you want to add a bit of crunch to your gazpacho, dice up some cucumber, peppers (red or green), fresh chives and mint to the soup.

Health Benefits

Tomatoes are the main ingredient in gazpacho, and as they are high in antioxidants, that equals great health benefits for you. Tomatoes contain the carotenoids beta-carotene and lycopene. These brightly coloured antioxidants have a vital role in helping to clean up free radicals in the blood system and from body tissues. Antioxidants are also beneficial to slowing down the signs of aging, together with being good for cardiovascular health.

Creamy Asparagus Soup

Ingredients

1 tbsp. olive oil
1 small onion
150g of asparagus
1 medium potato peeled and cubed (Maris Piper is best but any will do)
50ml of single cream
300ml of vegetable stock
Salt and freshly ground pepper to taste

Making It

1. Heat the olive oil in a saucepan. Add the onions and potato and fry over a gentle heat for about 5 minutes.
2. Take the tips off the asparagus and save them for step 3. Chop up the remaining asparagus in to 2cm length pieces. Place them in the saucepan together with the vegetable stock. Bring to the boil and then allow to simmer gently for about 25 minutes or until the asparagus is soft.
3. Whilst this is cooking, boil the asparagus tips in another saucepan, in some water, for about 10 minutes.
4. Allow the potato, onion and asparagus to cool to room temperature.
5. Pour into the Nutri Ninja and blend for about 30 seconds or until smooth. Add more stock or hot water if required.
6. Return the contents back to the saucepan and add the cooked asparagus tips, single cream and salt and pepper to taste. Gently reheat the soup before serving but do not allow to boil.

Health Benefits

Asparagus, a member of the lily family, is another ingredient loaded with nutrients. Asparagus contains vitamin K, folic acid, selenium, copper, vitamin C, vitamin B2 and vitamin E. Asparagus is a real power house at helping to fight disease. The high fibre is beneficial for a healthy bowel, as well as helping you to keep fuller for longer. Asparagus is rich in rutin, a natural substance found in plants. That, together with the vitamin C content, helps to protect the body from infection and boost energy levels. The iron levels found in asparagus means it is great for the immune system and preventing anaemia.

Pumpkin Soup

I love pumpkin soup, it is one of my favourites, especially with some freshly cooked bread to dunk in it. It also goes quite well with garlic bread.

Ingredients

1 tbsp. olive oil
200g of the flesh of a pumpkin, chopped
10g of butter
1 small onion, chopped
1 crushed garlic clove
1 pinch of ground cinnamon
350ml of vegetable stock
50ml of single cream
Salt and pepper to season

Making It

1. Heat the olive oil and butter in a saucepan and add the chopped onion. Cook for about 5 minutes over a gentle heat.
2. Add the garlic and pumpkin flesh and cook for another 5 minutes.
3. Add the vegetable stock.
4. Bring to the boil and then simmer for about 15 minutes, or until the pumpkin is soft.
5. Allow to cool to room temperature.
6. Place the contents in the Nutri Ninja and blend for about 30 seconds. Add more stock or hot water if required.
7. Return the contents to the saucepan and add the single cream. Gently reheat and serve.

Health Benefits

Pumpkins are a part of the Cucurbitaceae family, along with cucumbers and squash. Pumpkins contain no saturated fat or cholesterol. They are low in calories and high in antioxidants. Pumpkins are a great vegetable to use when trying to lose weight due to their high levels of dietary fibre. They are also packed with antioxidants, vitamins and minerals.

Pumpkins have incredibly high levels of vitamin A which is important for eye health, as well as being an anti-ageing nutrient that increases the production of collagen for smooth and younger looking skin.

Don't forget to save the seeds to munch on too. They are a fantastic source of dietary fibre and healthy fatty acids. They also contain high iron levels and zinc and selenium.

French Onion Soup

The smell of cooking onions is enough to make your taste buds tingle. French onion soup is really delicious and tastes perfect with some grilled French bread.

Ingredients

1 tbsp. of olive oil
2 medium onions
1 tbsp. flour
250ml of vegetable stock
1 garlic clove, crushed
2 tsp of Dijon mustard
Salt and freshly ground pepper to season

Making It

1. Heat the olive oil and fry the onions in a saucepan on a gentle heat until they are golden in colour, about 5 minutes.
2. Add the flour and cook for a further few seconds.
3. Add the vegetable stock, mustard and garlic.
4. Bring to the boil and then reduce the heat, simmering for about 15 minutes.
5. Allow to cool to room temperature (as per manufacturer's recommendation)
6. Pour the contents carefully in to the Nutri Ninja and blend for about 30 seconds, or until smooth. Add more stock or hot water if required.
7. Gently reheat before serving. Add salt and pepper to season if required.

Health Benefits

Onions, part of the allium family alongside garlic and leeks, should be a part of your diet on a regular basis. They are high in important flavonoids. When preparing onions, try not to take off too much of the outer layers. This is because a lot of the health benefits can be found here and peeling off too much will significantly reduce them. After chopping, try to leave the onion for about 5 minutes, it is thought to help enhance their health benefits.

The flavonoids found in onions are called quercetin. Quercetin is great for boosting the immune system. Onions also contain vitamin C, methionine, and cysteine which are all helpful for removing toxic heavy metals from the body. The sulphur compounds found in onions are good for improving red blood cell function and lowering cholesterol levels. Onions also help with lowering high blood pressure and promoting good blood circulation.

Thai Green Curry Soup

Ingredients
2 tbsp. olive oil
1 green chilli, chopped and deseeded
1 stick of lemongrass, chopped
1/2 onion, chopped
1 clove of garlic, crushed
1 teaspoon of ground cumin
1 teaspoon of ground coriander
1 tbsp. of Thai fish sauce
1 lime (zest and juice)
1 small chicken breast
400ml can of coconut milk
1 handful of fresh coriander leaves to garnish

Making It
1. In a saucepan fry the chopped onion in the olive oil for a few minutes.
2. Add the remaining ingredients except the coriander leaves, and bring to the boil. Simmer for about 10 to 15 minutes.
3. Whilst step 2 is cooking, fry the chopped chicken breast in a little olive oil until browned and cooked through.
4. Allow to cool to room temperature (as per manufacturer's instructions).
5. Pour the contents from step 2 into the Nutri Ninja and blend for about 30 seconds.
6. Return the contents to the saucepan and add the cooked chicken breast. Gently reheat until ready to serve.
Tip: You can make this into a full meal by adding it to some Basmati rice (or rice of your choice).

Health Benefits
Lemongrass features in many dishes from South East Asia. Aside from the flavour it adds to a soup, there are also health benefits including lowering cholesterol levels. The high levels of antioxidants found in lemongrass also help to fight other illnesses and diseases. Vitamin A can also be found in lemongrass which is beneficial for both eye and skin health.
Cumin is another popular ingredient from Asia, as well as Africa and Latin America. The taste is delicious and the health benefits are plentiful. Cumin is great for the immune system due to the vitamin C content, helping to fight coughs, colds and other viral infections. Cumin is very rich in iron which is beneficial to those prone to anaemia. The vitamin E is great for the premature signs of aging, helping the skin to stay young looking by acting as an antioxidant.
Coriander isn't just a pretty decorative garnish to put on dishes, it is a herb packed full with nutritional content. The health benefits include the clearing up of skin infections and inflammation such as eczema. Some of the acids present in coriander are useful for keeping cholesterol levels lower, particularly bad cholesterol. The high levels of iron are great for anaemia and research has shown that coriander can be useful in reducing blood pressure. Coriander is also rich in calcium, making it great for healthy bones.

Spicy Carrot and Lentil Soup

Ingredients

1 tbsp. of olive oil
3 large carrots
55g red lentils
3 tbsps. of coconut milk
20ml of single cream
1 small onion, chopped
250ml of vegetable stock
1 pinch of ground nutmeg
1 teaspoon of mild curry powder
Salt and freshly ground pepper to taste

Making It

1. Heat the olive oil in a saucepan and add the chopped onion, curry powder and nutmeg. Fry on a gentle heat for about 5 to 10 minutes. Don't allow the onion to burn.
2. Add the carrots and vegetable stock and bring to the boil. Turn the heat down and simmer on a gentle heat for about 15 minutes.
3. Allow to cool to room temperature as per the manufacturer's recommendations. Pour the contents in to the Nutri Ninja and blend for about 30 seconds. Add more stock or hot water if required.
4. Return the contents to the saucepan and add the red lentils. Bring to the boil and then simmer gently for about 15 minutes.
5. Add the single cream, coriander and coconut milk. Simmer for a further 5 minutes.
6. Add salt and freshly ground pepper to taste.

Health Benefits

Red lentils, from the legume family, are a great source of protein. They are high in fibre, making you feel fuller for longer. They are fat free and high in a range of nutrients. They have high levels of folic acid, essential for the nervous system and healthy blood cells. Lentils are also a good source of iron, and unlike red meat, do not contain the fat. Iron is vital for maintaining energy levels and is especially important for growing children and menstruating women.

Carrots are naturally sweet and high in fibre and carotenoids. The high fibre content is great for weight management, making you feel fuller for longer.

Even when nutmeg has been ground into a powder, it doesn't lose its fibre content. Nutmeg is said to be good for kidney and liver health by removing the build-up of toxins. The magnesium content is said to help stimulate the release of serotonin in the body which aids in sleep and relaxation.

Great Green Soup

Ingredients

1 tbsp. of olive oil
Small head of broccoli, chopped
1 small onion
1 courgette, chopped (if you use a smaller one, they are sweeter)
5 kale leaves
1 leek, chopped
1 celery stick, chopped
1 clove of garlic, crushed
350ml of vegetable stock
Add salt and freshly ground pepper

Making It

1. Heat the olive oil in a saucepan and add the chopped onion. Fry gently over a low heat for 2 to 3 minutes.
2. Add the crushed garlic and chopped leek and cook for a further 3 minutes.
3. Add the courgette, celery and kale, together with the vegetable stock.
4. Bring to the boil and then simmer for about 5 minutes.
5. Allow to cool to room temperature (as per the manufacturer's instructions).
6. Pour the contents into the Nutri Ninja and blend for about 30 seconds. Add more stock or hot water if required.
7. Reheat and serve.

Health Benefits

Broccoli is a great source of beta-carotene, calcium, vitamin C, potassium, magnesium and the vitamin B's. It is also full of dietary fibres which is great for making you feel full up and creating longer lasting energy.

Kale is an excellent source of vitamin K which helps to keep your blood healthy and aids in bone development. The high levels of vitamin A also help to keep your skin clear by maintaining a healthy skin cell function.

Courgettes are high in water content, but low in calories, so are great if you are watching your calorie intake. They contain potassium which is great for controlling blood pressure levels. They are high in fibre, making them ideal for the digestive system.

Coconut Chilli Soup

Ingredients

1 tbsp. olive oil
1 medium sweet potato, peeled and chopped
1/2 small red chilli, chopped and deseeded
400ml can of coconut milk
1/2 red onion
Salt and freshly ground pepper to season

Making It

1. Heat the olive oil in a saucepan and add the sweet potato, chilli and onion. Over a gentle heat, cook for around 10 minutes.
2. Add the coconut milk and simmer for a further 10 minutes.
3. Allow to cool to room temperature.
4. Pour the contents into the Nutri Ninja and blend for about 30 seconds. Add hot water if a thinner consistency is required.
5. Gently reheat when you are ready to serve. Season with salt and pepper to taste.

Health Benefits

Coconut milk is a great alternative to milk, and is also highly nutritious. Coconuts are rich in iron, sodium, selenium, calcium, magnesium, phosphorous, fibre, vitamins B1, B3, B5 B 6 and C & E. Coconut milk is high in saturated fats but it is much healthier than other saturated fat products. Lauric acid is the main saturated fat found in coconut milk, which is said to help promote brain development and bone health. Just check on the carton/tin before buying to make sure there are no added extras to the milk. Even better, why not try making your own?

Sweet Potatoes are high in beta-carotene, vitamin A and vitamin C. The vitamin A can help support healthy blood cell development.

Chillis not only taste good, they also speed up your metabolism. They raise your endorphin levels making you feel better.

Red Onions can really boost your health. They contain many minerals and vitamins which help keep your body at optimum health levels. They contain folate, potassium, magnesium and vitamins B-6, C & K.

Curried Banana

Ingredients

1 tbsp. olive oil
1 clove garlic, crushed
1 small onion, chopped
1 tablespoon of mild curry powder
300ml of vegetable stock
50ml of single cream
1 ripe banana
1 lime

Making It

1. Heat the oil in a saucepan and gently cook the onion and garlic on a low heat for about 10 minutes.
2. Add the curry powder and cook whilst stirring for a further 2 or 3 minutes.
3. Add the vegetable stock, chopped banana and juice of the lime. Bring to the boil, and then reduce heat and simmer for about 5-10 minutes.
4. Allow to cool to room temperature.
5. Pour contents into the Nutri Ninja. Stir in the cream and blend for about 30 seconds or until smooth. Add more stock or hot water if required.
6. Add any salt or pepper, if required. Gently reheat before serving.

Health Benefits

Bananas are high in potassium, making them great for lowering blood pressure. The natural sweet taste of a banana can help curb those with a sweet tooth, whilst leaving you feeling full, due to the high fibre levels they contain.

Curry powder contains turmeric, a very powerful spice that is said to help a variety of conditions, owing to its anti-inflammatory benefits. It is bright yellow to look at and tastes warm and peppery.

Classic Chicken Soup

Ingredients
1 tbsp. of olive oil
1 medium onion, chopped
1 garlic clove, crushed
350ml of chicken stock
1 medium potato, chopped into cubes (Maris Piper is best but any will do)
75g cooked chicken breast, shredded
50ml single cream (optional)
Salt and freshly ground pepper to season

Making It
1. Heat the olive oil in a saucepan and add the chopped onions and crushed garlic. Cook over a gentle heat for about 3 minutes.
2. Add the potato and cooked for a further 3 minutes.
3. Add the chicken stock and bring to the boil.
4. Reduce the heat and allow to simmer for about 10 minutes.
5. Allow to cool to room temperature.
6. Pour the contents into the Nutri Ninja and blend for about 30 seconds or until smooth. Add more stock or hot water if required.
7. Return to the saucepan and add the shredded chicken breast. Stir in the optional single cream. Heat gently for about 5 minutes.
8. Season with salt and freshly ground pepper if required. Serve and enjoy!

Health Benefits
Chicken has many health benefits including protein, essential vitamins and minerals. Protein is an essential part of our diet, helping to build and repair muscle. The B vitamins found in chicken are great for boosting immunity and helping with skin conditions. Chicken soup is not only a tasty and comforting soup when suffering from a cold or sore throat, it also provides some relief.

Cauliflower Cheese

Ingredients

1 tbsp. olive oil
1 small onion, chopped
1 medium potato, chopped (Maris Piper if possible)
1 small cauliflower, broken into small florets
300ml vegetable stock
100ml semi skimmed milk
75g grated cheddar cheese (mature/vintage)
Salt and freshly ground pepper to taste

Making It

1. Heat the olive oil in the saucepan and add the chopped onions. Cook on a gentle heat for a few minutes.
2. Add the chopped potato and cook for a further few minutes, again on a gentle heat.
3. Add the vegetable stock and cauliflower and bring to the boil. Reduce the heat and allow to simmer for about 15 minutes or until the vegetables are soft.
4. Allow the contents to cool to room temperature.
5. Pour the contents into the Nutri Ninja and blend for about 30 seconds. Add more stock or hot water if required.
6. Return the contents to the saucepan. Add the milk and the Cheddar cheese. Over a gentle heat, stir until the cheese has melted. If you prefer a richer taste, add more cheese. Don't allow the soup to boil.
7. Season with salt and freshly ground pepper if desired.
8. Serve and enjoy!

Health Benefits

Cauliflower is a great source of choline, an essential nutrient for memory and learning. It also has a high fibre content which is beneficial for a healthy digestive system and aids with weight loss by making you feel fuller for longer. Cauliflower is also a great source of vitamin C.

Cheddar cheese may be high in fat and calories, but if eaten in moderation, is a very beneficial source of protein and calcium, essential for your diet. Plus, it tastes delicious in a soup!

Pea, Bacon and Cheese

Ingredients

1 tbsp. olive oil

1 generous tbsp. of butter

4 rashers of bacon, chopped

1 small onion

350ml of vegetable stock

1 carrot, grated

1 small leek, chopped

75g of peas (fresh or frozen)

75g of grated cheese (Cheddar is fine, or your own favourite)

1 pinch of ground nutmeg

Making It

1. In a frying pan, heat the olive oil and add the chopped bacon. Fry on a gentle heat until the bacon is crispy. Place the bacon on a piece of kitchen roll and put to one side.
2. Melt the butter in a saucepan and add the chopped onion and leek. Cook on a gentle heat for about 10 minutes.
3. Add the vegetable stock, grated carrot and pinch of nutmeg. Bring to the boil and then simmer on a gentle heat for about 10 minutes, or until the vegetables are soft.
4. Allow the contents to cool to room temperature.
5. Pour the contents into the Nutri Ninja and blend for about 30 seconds or until smooth. Add more stock or hot water if required.
6. Return contents to the saucepan and add the bacon and peas. Simmer on a gentle heat for about 5 minutes.
7. Add the grated cheese and stir until melted. Keep the heat on low to avoid boiling.
8. Season with salt and freshly ground pepper if required.

Health Benefits

Leeks are part of the onion and garlic family and offer a great array of health benefits. Leeks are high in the antioxidant polyphenol and the flavonoid kaempferol, which play a part in protecting our blood vessels and cells from damage. The allicin found in leeks can help fight dangerous free radicals in your body. Leeks are also low in calories yet help to make you feel full. Leeks also contain high levels of vitamin K and A.

Peas are low in calories and high in fibre, making them a great addition to any weight loss or maintenance plan. Peas are also high in lutein, a carotenoid vitamin that is fantastic for keeping eyes healthy. Peas have a high iron content, essential for keeping energy levels at optimum level and to help with concentration.

Cheddar cheese may be high in fat and calories, but if eaten in moderation, is a very beneficial source of protein and calcium, essential for your diet. Plus, it tastes delicious in a soup!

Carrots are naturally sweet and high in fibre and carotenoids. The high fibre content is great for weight management, making you feel fuller for longer.

Even when nutmeg has been ground into a powder, it doesn't lose its fibre content. Nutmeg is said to be good for kidney and liver health by removing the build-up of toxins. The magnesium content is said to help stimulate the release of serotonin in the body which aids in sleep and relaxation.

Parsnip, Parmesan and Chilli

Ingredients

1 tbsp. of olive oil
1 small onion
1 clove of garlic, crushed
3 medium parsnips, chopped
50g parmesan cheese
1 small red chilli, chopped and deseeded
350ml of vegetable stock
Salt and freshly ground pepper to taste

Making It

1. Heat the oil in a saucepan and add the chopped onions. Cook on a gentle heat for a few minutes. Add the crushed garlic and cook for a further few minutes.
2. Add the chopped parsnips. Cook gently for a further 2 to 3 minutes.
3. Add the vegetable stock and chopped chilli and bring to the boil. Turn the heat down and add the parmesan cheese. Gently simmer for about 15-20 minutes, or until the parsnips are soft.
4. Allow the contents to cool to room temperature.
5. Add the contents to your Nutri Ninja and blend for about 30 seconds. Add more stock or hot water if required.
6. Reheat gently when ready to serve. Season with salt and pepper if required.

Health Benefits

Parsnips add a welcome sweet taste to any soup dish. They offer a wide variety of health benefits owing to their levels of potassium, vitamin C, fibre content and folate. Thanks to the high potassium and folate levels, parsnips are particularly good for heart health. Parsnips are low in calories and high in fibre so can contribute to weight loss and maintenance.

Chillis not only taste good, they also speed up your metabolism. They raise your endorphin levels making you feel better.

Although Parmesan cheese should be eaten in moderation, like most cheeses, it is a good source of protein and calcium, both essential for growth and development. Parmesan cheese is also easier to digest than many other cheeses due to the aging process (which allows the protein to get broken down prior to digestion). The cholesterol content of Parmesan cheese is also lower than other cheeses, making it a preferable choice.

Chicken and Chorizo Soup

Ingredients

2 tbsp. olive oil

1/2 medium onion, chopped

1 carrot, chopped

Half chicken breast, cut into small pieces

1 garlic clove, crushed

1 parsnip, chopped

350ml chicken stock

1 chorizo sausage, finely chopped

Making It

1. Heat 1tbsp of the oil in a saucepan. Add the chopped onion and gently cook for a few minutes.
2. Add the carrot, parsnip and crushed garlic and continue to cook on a low heat for a further 3 or 4 minutes.
3. Add the chicken stock and bring to the boil.
4. Reduce the heat and simmer for about 10 to 15 minutes or until the vegetables are tender.
5. During this time add the other tbsp. of olive oil to a frying pan and heat. Add the sliced chicken and fry over a gentle heat for about 5 minutes. Add the sliced chorizo and continue to cook both the chicken and chorizo for a further 5 minutes, or until cooked through.
6. Allow to cool to room temperature.
7. Pour the contents from the saucepan (vegetables and chicken stock) in to the Nutri Ninja and blend for about 30 seconds or until smooth. Add more stock or hot water if required.
8. Return the contents to the saucepan and add the cooked chicken and chorizo. Simmer gently on a low heat for about 5 minutes.
9. Add a little salt and freshly ground pepper if required.

Health Benefits

Chicken has many health benefits including protein, essential vitamins and minerals. Protein is an essential part of our diet, helping to build and repair muscle. The B vitamins found in chicken are great for boosting immunity and helping with skin conditions. Chicken soup is not only a tasty and comforting soup when suffering from a cold or sore throat, it also provides some relief.

Parsnips add a welcome sweet taste to any soup dish. They offer a wide variety of health benefits owing to their levels of potassium, vitamin C, fibre content and folate. Thanks to the high potassium and folate levels, parsnips are particularly good for heart health. Parsnips are low in calories and high in fibre so can contribute to weight loss and maintenance.

Carrots are naturally sweet and high in fibre and carotenoids. The high fibre content is great for weight management, making you feel fuller for longer.

Chorizo, although very tasty, should be eaten in moderation. It contains a lot of fat and sodium, neither of which are good for you. However, when included occasionally in your diet, it does benefit from a rich source of selenium and zinc. Protein can also be found in chorizo which assists with repairing and developing muscle tissue.

Tomato and Red Pepper Soup

Ingredients

2 tbsp. of olive oil
1 medium red pepper, halved and deseeded
6 ripe tomatoes, skinned and halved
1 medium onion, chopped
1 garlic clove, crushed
1 tbsp. of fresh basil, chopped
350ml of vegetable stock
Salt and freshly ground pepper to taste

Making It

1. Preheat the oven to 190C (375 F) or gas mark 5.
2. Place the red pepper and tomatoes on a baking tray and drizzle with 1 tbsp. of olive oil. Sprinkle with the chopped basil. Add salt and freshly ground black pepper if required.
3. Bake in the oven for 1 hour.
4. Heat 1 tbsp. of olive oil in a saucepan and cook the onion and garlic for a few minutes. Turn the heat down really low and cover and cook gently for about 5 to 10 minutes.
5. When the red pepper and tomatoes have finished in the oven, add them to the saucepan, together with the vegetable stock. Bring to the boil.
6. Allow to cool to room temperature.
7. Pour the contents in to the Nutri Ninja and blend for about 30 seconds or until smooth. Add more stock or hot water if required.
8. Reheat gently. Serve and enjoy!

Health Benefits

Red peppers contain the highest amount of vitamin C out of all the bell peppers, which is fantastic for your immune system to help keep your skin looking clear and healthy. They are rich in beta-carotene and capsaicin. Capsaicin is great for easing inflammation and reducing bad cholesterol. Red peppers are very high in vitamin A and E, which is beneficial for healthy skin and hair. As a bonus, they are also very low in calories and taste great.

Tomatoes are high in antioxidants, which equals great health benefits for you. Tomatoes contain the carotenoids beta-carotene and lycopene. These brightly coloured antioxidants have a vital role in helping to clean up free radicals in the blood system and from body tissues. Antioxidants are also beneficial to slowing down the signs of aging, together with being good for cardiovascular health.

Spicy Parsnip Soup

Ingredients

1 tbsp. of olive oil
2 small parsnips, chopped
350ml of vegetable stock
1 small onion, chopped
1 clove of garlic, crushed
2 teaspoons of mild curry powder (or a mix of ground cumin, turmeric, coriander and garam masala)
1/2 inch of fresh root ginger, finely chopped or grated

Making It

1. Heat the oil in a saucepan and add the onion and garlic. Gently cook on a low heat for about 10 minutes.
2. Add the curry powder and ginger and cook for a further 3 minutes, stirring continuously.
3. Add the vegetable stock and chopped parsnips. Bring to the boil for a minute and then reduce heat to simmer for around 25 minutes or until the parsnips are tender.
4. Allow the contents to cool to room temperature (as per manufacturer's instructions).
5. Pour the contents into the Nutri Ninja and blend for about 30 seconds or until smooth. Add more stock or hot water if required.
6. Reheat on a gentle heat when ready to eat. Season with salt and freshly ground pepper if required. Serve and enjoy!

For a slight variation you can add a peeled and chopped pear at the blending stage to add a little sweetness to the mix. It tastes really great.

Health Benefits

Parsnips are from the carrot family and have the same lovely sweetness to them. Nutritionally, parsnips help to strengthen hair and nails. The potassium, sulphur, silicon, chlorine, vitamin C and phosphorus all help to improve the quality of the skin, helping with any skin disorders and generally benefitting the skin. Parsnips are another vegetable that are high in fibre and low in calories, making them great for maintaining a healthy weight, or as part of a weight loss program.

Premade curry powders will vary as to what spices are included, but they will all contain valuable health benefits including boosting the immune system, acting as a detoxifier and preventing heart problems. Turmeric contains anti-inflammatory benefits, helping ease joint pain and arthritic symptoms. Turmeric is also beneficial for bone health, strengthening and protecting them.

Broccoli and Stilton Soup

Ingredients

1 tbsp. of olive oil
25g of butter
1 clove of garlic, crushed
1 small leek, chopped
1 small potato (Maris Piper is best but any type will be ok)
200g of broccoli florets
350ml of vegetable stock
75g of Stilton cheese
50ml of double cream

Making It

1. Heat the butter and olive oil in a saucepan and add the potato, garlic and leek. Cook gently on a low heat for about 10 minutes or until soft.
2. Add the broccoli and vegetable stock and bring to the boil. Reduce heat and simmer for about 8 minutes or until the broccoli is tender but not overcooked.
3. Add the Stilton and stir in until it is almost melted. Add the cream.
4. Allow to cool to room temperature (according to the manufacturer's instructions).
5. Pour the contents in to the Nutri Ninja and blend until smooth. Add more stock or hot water if required.
6. Gently reheat when ready to eat. Season with salt and freshly ground pepper if required.
7. Serve and enjoy!

Health Benefits

Broccoli should be a staple in everyone's diet due to its supreme health benefits. Broccoli is a good source of fibre and is low in calories. It is also rich in beta-carotene, folic acid, calcium, vitamin B, potassium and magnesium. The vitamin K present in broccoli makes it great for bone health. There is enough vitamin C in just one cup of broccoli to meet the daily recommended intake - making this powerful vegetable essential for healthy looking skin and a strong immune system. Broccoli is also incredibly high in protein, which is where most of the calories come from, unlike meat where the protein comes mainly from fat. Past studies have shown that broccoli has powerful healing properties, with cancer fighting substances contained within it.

Stilton is a traditional English blue cheese made from cow's milk. It contains numerous health benefits, owing to the probiotic content found within it. The probiotics help to improve the health of your digestive tract. Lactobacillus is a common type of probiotic which is found in Stilton cheese. It helps to make an unwelcoming environment for harmful bacteria. It also helps to breakdown the food within your body.

Mushroom Soup

Ingredients

1tbsp of olive oil
1tbsp or about 10g of butter
1 small onion, chopped
1 garlic clove, crushed
1 small carrot, chopped
75g of sliced mushrooms (chestnut work well)
75g of sliced shiitake mushrooms
1 tbsp. of chopped fresh rosemary, or 1 tsp of ground rosemary
350ml of vegetable stock
Handful of grated parmesan cheese to sprinkle on top (optional)

Making It

1. Heat the olive oil in a saucepan and add the onion and garlic. Gently cook on a low heat for about 5 minutes.
2. Add the vegetable stock, the chestnut mushrooms (or mushroom of your choice), and the rosemary. Bring to the boil and then simmer on a gentle heat for about 10 minutes.
3. Allow to cool to room temperature (as per manufacturer's instructions).
4. Pour the contents in to the Nutri Ninja and blend for about 30 seconds or until smooth. Add more stock or hot water if required.
5. In a frying pan, heat the butter. Add the shiitake mushrooms and gently fry for about 5 minutes, until they begin to brown.
6. Return the contents from the Nutri Ninja to the saucepan and add the fried mushrooms. Gently reheat.
7. Season with salt and freshly ground pepper if required.
8. Serve in to bowls. Sprinkle parmesan cheese over the top if you want to. Enjoy!

Health Benefits

Mushrooms are fat free, low in calories and rich in minerals. Shiitake mushrooms, according to some Japanese studies, are said to help lower cholesterol and blood pressure. They are also recommended for anti-aging and general vitality of health. Mushrooms are good sources of selenium, a mineral that helps to protect our cells from damage that may lead to chronic illnesses. Mushrooms are also a source of vitamin D, so eating them is a good way to up your levels.

Rosemary is rich in folic acid, vitamin A, vitamin C, potassium, calcium, iron, magnesium, copper and manganese. Who would have thought this humble herb could pack such a positive health punch? Rosemary is good for the immune system, the digestive system and increasing circulation. Rosemary is also said to improve concentration by increasing the blood flow to the brain.

Carrot and Coriander Soup

Ingredients

1 tbsp of olive oil
1 clove of garlic, crushed
3 medium carrots, chopped
1 small carrot, grated
350ml of vegetable stock
2 tbsp of fresh coriander, chopped
1 tsp of freshly ground nutmeg or ground nutmeg
50ml of single cream (optional)

Making It

1. Heat the olive oil in a saucepan and add the onion and crushed garlic. Cook gently for about 5 minutes without browning.
2. Add the vegetable stock, chopped carrots and nutmeg. Bring to the boil and then simmer gently for about 10 minutes or until the vegetables are tender.
3. Allow to cool to room temperature (according to manufacturer's instructions).
4. Pour the contents into the Nutri Ninja and blend for about 30 seconds or until smooth. Add more stock or hot water if required.
5. Gently reheat the soup when ready to eat.
6. Serve the soup into bowls and sprinkle the grated carrot and fresh coriander on top. Add the cream now if you want to.
7. Season with salt and freshly ground pepper if required.
8. Enjoy!

Health Benefits

Coriander isn't just a pretty decorative garnish to put on dishes, it is a herb packed full with nutritional content. The health benefits include the clearing up of skin infections and inflammation such as eczema. Some of the acids present in coriander are useful for keeping cholesterol levels lower, particularly bad cholesterol. The high levels of iron are great for anaemia and research has shown that coriander can be useful in reducing blood pressure. Coriander is also rich in calcium, making it great for healthy bones.

Carrots make them the perfect ingredient for a nice warming soup. They are high in fibre and low in calories. They are a great detoxifier, boosting the health of the liver and digestive system. It is true that carrots help with eye health, due to the wide range of carotenoids found in them. Carrots are rich in vitamin A which helps your body to produce rhodopsin, a purple pigment that helps you to see in dim light.

Pea and Mint Soup

Ingredients
1 tbsp of olive oil
1 small onion, chopped
1 clove of garlic, crushed
1 medium potato (Maris Piper is a good choice)
350ml of vegetable stock
75g of fresh green peas, shelled (if they are not in season then frozen peas can be used)
A few mint leaves, shredded
50ml of single cream (optional)

Making It
1. Heat the oil in a saucepan and add the onions and garlic. Cook on a gentle heat for a few minutes until soft, do not brown.
2. Add the chopped potato and stock. Simmer for about 10 minutes or until the potato is soft.
3. Add the peas and mint leaves. Simmer for 5 more minutes.
4. Allow the contents to cool to room temperature.
5. Pour the contents into the Nutri Ninja and blend for about 3o seconds or until smooth. Add more stock or hot water if required.
6. Stir in the single cream if required.
7. Season with salt and freshly ground pepper if desired.
8. Serve and enjoy!

Health Benefits
Peas are a staple in many people's diets. What isn't always appreciated about the humble pea though, is the amount of nutrition that is packed into something so small. Peas are low in fat yet high in fibre, protein and micronutrients. Peas are also high in antioxidants and anti-inflammatory properties, which is said to be great for reducing the risk of heart disease, cancer, Alzheimer's and other age related illnesses. Peas are also good for your bones, owing to the high levels of vitamin k present.
Mint stimulates the digestive enzymes which can help convert fat in to useable energy. Mint is an ancient herb that has been used for medicinal purposes for hundreds of years. The benefits of mint include aiding digestion and reducing nausea.

Beetroot and Rhubarb

Ingredients

1 tbsp of olive oil
1/2 medium onion, chopped
1 clove of garlic, crushed
1/2 cm of finely chopped or grated fresh root ginger
1 small peeled raw beetroot (or beet!)
100g rhubarb, chopped
350ml of vegetable stock

Making It

1. Heat the olive oil in the saucepan and add the onions and garlic. Gently cook for about 5 minutes without browning.
2. Add the ginger and cook for a further 30 seconds.
3. Add the vegetable stock and rhubarb. Bring to the boil and then reduce the heat. Simmer for about 5 minutes or until the rhubarb is soft.
4. In a separate pan boil the beetroot for about 20 minutes or until soft.
5. Allow to cool to room temperature (as per manufacturer's instructions).
6. Pour all the contents into the Nutri Ninja and blend for about 30 seconds or until smooth. The texture of the beetroot might mean the soup is quite thick - feel free to add water to thin it some more.
7. Reheat when ready to eat, on a gentle heat. Season with salt and freshly ground pepper if required.

Health Benefits

Ginger is great for nausea and unsettled stomachs. Ginger is thought to be good at aiding digestion by making the stomach empty more quickly and effectively. This is useful for those who suffer with the uncomfortable symptoms of indigestion. The spice is also a known natural remedy for colds and symptoms of the flu.

Beetroot is rich in iron, an essential mineral required for healthy blood and energy production. Beetroot widens the blood vessels, allowing oxygen to flow more easily, increasing stamina and energy levels. Beetroot has about 20 times the amount of nitrates as other vegetables. The nitrate converts into nitric oxide in our bodies, this provides our bodies with longer lasting energy. The betacyanin found in beetroot (the pigment that gives beetroot its bright purple colour), is thought to reduce the risk of the development of some types of cancer. The high fibre content of beetroots is great for a healthy bowel function.

Rhubarb is high in fibre and low in calories, making it great for health weight loss and maintenance. The many compounds found in rhubarb mean that it can help speed up metabolism and burn fat at a faster rate. The high fibre content means consuming rhubarb will help with digestion. Rhubarb is also very high in vitamin K, a very significant ingredient for optimal brain health and bone protection.

Making Stock

All the soup recipes in this book include a stock of some kind, as the base.

You can buy supermarket made stock, there is a huge range of both fresh and dried options available.

However, if you would like to make your own then it is easy enough to do, plus, you know exactly what is in it and adjust the flavour according to your taste.

Vegetable Stock

This recipe will make about 1 litre. If you want to make more or less, you can adjust the ingredients accordingly.

Ingredients

1 bay leaf
1 clove of garlic, crushed
1 teaspoon of peppercorns
3 small carrots, chopped
2 sticks of celery, chopped
1 medium leek, chopped
1/2 onion, chopped
1 tbsp. olive oil

Making It

1. Heat the olive oil in a large saucepan. Add the onion, leek and carrot and cook on a low heat for about 2 to 3 minutes.
2. Pour enough water (about 1and a half litres) to generously cover the vegetables.
3. Turn the heat up and add the garlic, peppercorn, celery and bay leaf. Bring to the boil and cook gently for about 15 minutes.
4. Turn the heat down and simmer for a further 30 minutes.
5. Sieve the mixture, discarding the vegetables (or find another use for them).
6. Use the stock for your soup, or store in a sealed container until ready to use. The stock can keep in the fridge for about 3 days or can be frozen in batches for future use.

Feel free to vary the vegetables according to what you have available, and your own personal preferences. A dash of ginger often adds a nice flavour to the stock too.

Chicken Stock

Ingredients

Chicken (roasted or unroasted) carcass including legs, wings and bones.
3 litres of water
3 small carrots, chopped
1 medium onion, chopped
1 tablespoon of whole black peppercorns, crushed
1 leek, chopped
2 sticks of celery, chopped
2 garlic cloves, crushed
2 bay leaves

Making It

1.   Place all of the above ingredients in a large pan or stockpot.
2.   Pour in enough water to cover all the chicken and ingredients.
3.   Turn the heat on and bring to the boil. Turn the heat down and gently simmer for 2 to 3 hours. Make sure you skim the top every half an hour, or as required, with a large spoon.
4.   Strain the stock and either use straight away, or store for future use. The stock will keep in the fridge for a few days, or it can be frozen.

BONUS - Homemade Crouton Recipes

Croutons are cheap and easy enough to buy from the supermarket, but nothing quite beats the satisfying feeling of having cooked them yourself. You know exactly what is going in them, and you can experiment with a variety of different ingredients, creating some delicious tastes. What's more, they are really easy to make.

Making Croutons

Croutons can either be toasted in a frying pan or in the oven.

Croutons are easy to freeze so you can make more than you need and defrost as and when you need them. Just pop the ones you want to freeze in a sealable plastic food bag.

Croutons can be stored in an airtight container for a few days.

The best kind of bread to use is slightly stale bread, but you can use fresh bread, whatever you have handy.

You can use any kind of bread; white, wholemeal, French bread etc.

Many recipes recommend cutting off the crust when making croutons. I actually quite like to leave it on, it adds extra flavour and texture. But it is entirely up to you.

How you cut and shape your croutons is your own choice. You can go for a rustic, ununiformed shape, or make them more cube like.

You can use either butter or oil to coat them in. Butter tends to cook more quickly so you will have to keep a closer eye on them when they are cooking so that they don't burn. Butter also gives a more creamy taste when the croutons are mixed in with the soup.

You can experiment with adding extra herbs, garlic, spices and so on, to add some extra flavour. Use the following recipe for your base, adjusting and replacing as you wish.

Classic Croutons

Half a loaf of slightly stale bread (either sliced sandwich bread, French baguette, or another choice).

Half a cup of melted butter, olive oil, or a combination of both.

Making Them

I prefer to cook mine in the oven, but you can cook them using a frying pan. Just ensure that you turn them frequently so they don't burn, and use enough oil or butter to cook them in.

1. Preheat the oven to 190C (375F) or gas mark 5.

2. Cut the bread according to the kind of croutons you want. For classic crouton cubes use the sliced sandwich bread and cut into cubes, about an inch in length. For any other kind of bread you could create a more rustic type by just tearing small chunks off. With the baguette you can cut off thin slices, about a half inch in thickness, or less.

3. On a lightly greased baking tray place the croutons. Lightly coat each one with the butter or oil, using a brush if you have one. Be sure to cover each side.

4. Place them in the oven for about 10 minutes cooking time. Take them out half way through to shake them about a bit and make sure each side is toasted. When they are browned they are ready. Remember to keep a close eye on them so they don't burn.

Recipe Variations

Garlic Croutons - Add one crushed or finely grated garlic clove to the oil or butter before coating the croutons. The further in advance you are able to do this, the stronger the garlic taste will be.

Spicy Croutons - You can choose which spice you want to add, I quite like to use ground cayenne pepper (about 2 to 3 pinches) but you can also try mild curry powder, turmeric, paprika etc. Just add the spices in to the butter or oil before coating the bread.

Cheesy Croutons - Cheesy croutons are absolutely delicious in soup. Use grated parmesan cheese (about a 1/4 of a cup in the above recipe). Sprinkle the cheese over the croutons about half way through the cooking, when you take them out to shake them about.

Naan Croutons - Cut the naan bread up in to small cubes and fry in a little oil until brown all over. Remove from the heat and drain away any excess oil. Add some sesame seeds and heat for about 20 seconds until golden brown.

SAUCES, DIPS & SPREADS RECIPE BOOK

Using a Nutri Ninja

We've had our Nutri Ninja for well over a year now and it gets used almost every day. It only takes up a little space and is so versatile we can use it for creating all kinds of healthy eating recipes.

In the beginning we only used to make smoothies (you can see these in Nutri Ninja Recipe Book – 70 Smoothie Recipes for Weight Loss, Increased Energy and Improved Health) but then we started to experiment with other foods.

Now we make a variety of healthy meals including soups, sauces, dips, nut butters, frozen yoghurts and other really tasty desserts!

The great thing is, we know exactly what is going in each time. No more wondering what a certain 'ingredient' is listed on the packaging.

Most of the recipes in this book are really very straight forward – I've tried to keep them as simple as possible. I'm more about the tasting of what we make so I'm keen to get to it as soon as I can!

Aside from the delicious taste of these homemade sauces, dips, butters and desserts, the recipes also offer a huge amount of nutritional health benefits. I have tried to list as many of those benefits where I can under each recipe.

Which Blender?

The recipes in this book are aimed at all high power blenders. We personally use the Nutri Ninja BL450, but they can also be used in the Nutri Ninja Professional IQ BL480, the popular Nutribullet or any high powered blender.

Using the Nutri Ninja Blender

Always refer to the manufacturer's manual that came with your Nutri Ninja. Some recipes within this book will require cooking. Always allow the contents to cool to room temperature before placing in your Nutri Ninja cup. Never fill the cups above the 'MAX' line.

A note about blending dry ingredients. The manufacturers advise to always add liquid when blending dry ingredients such as seeds and nuts.

Equipment

Aside from the Nutri Ninja blender (or other high powered blender like a Nutribullet or Vitamix), you shouldn't really need much more than what is already in your kitchen;
Saucepan/frying pan
Kitchen scales
Measuring cup
Garlic crusher
Grater

Preparing the Ingredients

I have only used ingredients that I have been able to source from my local supermarket or health food store. We want to keep things simple so that we don't get disheartened and stop using the blender!

Depending on which recipes you make, you will need a variety of herbs and spices. These can keep for a long periods of time and be used across many different recipes, not only in these recipes but also in other meals you cook. So, consider them an investment if you don't already have them.

SAUCES, DIPS & DRESSINGS

We have really enjoyed experimenting with our favourite sauces, dips and dressings in the Nutri Ninja.

Most of our sauces serve 4 people. They can of course be doubled up or halved, depending on your needs.

Our dips and dressings are usually enough for 4 people to enjoy. Each recipe should yield a ramekin bowl size quantity, averaging about 150 to 200ml.

Plum & Honey Dip

This sweet dip tastes lovely with duck. We especially like dunking duck spring rolls in it. Yum.

Ingredients

170g plums
5tbsp honey
2tbsp lemon juice
1tbsp (15g) chopped onion
½ tsp lemon zest
½ tsp (8g) grated ginger
Pinch salt
Pinch ground cloves

Making It

Place all the ingredients in a saucepan and bring to the boil over a medium heat. Lower the heat and simmer for about 10 to 15 minutes or until the plums are stewed.

Allow to cool to room temperature. Place in the Nutri Ninja blender and blend until smooth, about 20 to 30 seconds.

If you prefer the sauce to be a little sweeter, add some more honey now and blend again.

Health Benefits

Plums are low in calories and contain no saturated fats. They are high in potassium and have a low glycemic index.

Caramelised Onion Gravy

Serves 4

This onion gravy goes really well with sausage and mash.

Ingredients

60ml olive oil

2 large onions, finely chopped

4 garlic cloves, peeled and crushed

1 teaspoon paprika

400ml chicken or vegetable stock

Salt and pepper to season

Making It

1.　Heat the oil in a large sauce pan over a medium heat. Add the chopped onions and cook for about 30 minutes, stirring often, until soft.

2.　Add in the garlic and paprika. Cook for a further 5 minutes.

3.　Add the stock and bring to the boil. Reduce to a simmer and cook gently for a further 5 minutes.

4.　Allow to cool to room temperature and then add to the Nutri Ninja blender. Blend for about 20 to 30 seconds or until smooth.

5.　When you are ready to use the gravy, reheat it over a low heat until hot. Season with salt and pepper if required.

Health Benefits

Onions are part of the allium family of vegetables along with garlic and leeks. They are great for strengthening your immune system and combatting infection. Onions are also rich in flavonoids which can help protect you from heart disease.

Honey and Mustard Sauce

Serves 4

Honey and mustard is a deliciously sweet sauce that goes well with oven roasted or stir fried chicken breasts.

Ingredients

75g chopped onions
1 small carrot (approx. 50g), peeled & sliced
2 cloves of garlic, peeled & crushed
1tsp Dijon mustard
4tbsp honey
4tbsp single cream
100ml water (approx.)

Making It

1. Prepare all the ingredients and place everything into the Nutri Ninja blender, but leave out the cream.
2. Blend for about 20 to 30 seconds. You will need to blend it in short bursts and keep stopping to scrape the sides down.
3. Depending on the consistency, you may need to add a little extra water, but be careful not to add too much (not only will you make it too thin, you will also lose a lot of the taste).
4. Whilst you are cooking your meat or fish, pour the sauce into a saucepan and gently heat. As you are heating it slowly stir in the single cream. Gently simmer until the sauce is hot. Add more cream if you require a thicker consistency.
5. Pour over your meat/fish and enjoy!

Roasted Red Pepper Dip

Roasted Red Pepper Dip makes a fantastic starter served with a selection of raw vegetables.

Ingredients

2 sweet red peppers
1 garlic clove, peeled
1tbsp lemon juice
2tsp olive oil
25g fresh white breadcrumbs
Salt and black pepper to season (optional)

Making It

1. Preheat the oven to 200c (gas mark 6). Halve and seed the red peppers. Place on a baking tray with the garlic clove.
2. Cook for about 20 minutes or until the peppers and garlic are soft.
3. Allow to cool to room temperature. Add to the Nutri Ninja blender together with the lemon juice and olive oil.
4. Blend for about 20 seconds, or until smooth.
5. Stir in the breadcrumbs.
6. Season with salt/pepper if required.

Health Benefits

Red peppers are low in calories, rich in dietary fibre and also an excellent source of vitamins A, C, and E. Red peppers are a good source of iron so beneficial for people suffering with anaemia.

Barbecue Sauce

There are many ways to make BBQ sauce, and there are many ways to eat it! We find this way really straight forward and the sun dried tomatoes give it a lovely rich flavour. You can make this as a sauce to pour over meats or vegetables, or make it thicker to use as a dip.

Ingredients

100g sun dried tomatoes
2tbsp olive oil
2tbsp apple cider vinegar
2tsp paprika
2tsp cumin
2tsp chilli powder
2tsp garlic powder
400ml water

Making It

1. Soak the sun dried tomatoes in 200ml of the water until soft (about 30 minutes).
2. Add the soft tomatoes together with the water to the Nutri Ninja blender.
3. Add all the remaining ingredients.
4. Blend for about 20 to 30 seconds or until smooth. Add the remaining 200ml of water gradually until you get to a thinner more sauce like consistency. If you are making it as a dip don't add too much water.
5. If you are using it as a sauce to pour over food heat it up in a sauce pan on a gentle heat for about 10 minutes until warmed through.

Health Benefits

Sun dried tomatoes are rich in iron and vitamins C and K.

Simple Tomato Pasta Sauce

Serves 4

This sauce is very adaptable for adding to many different dishes. It goes perfectly with pasta or added to minced beef for a Spaghetti Bolognese.

Ingredients

400g chopped tomatoes (tinned or fresh)
1 small onion, chopped (about 100g)
4tbsp tomato puree
2 garlic cloves, peeled and crushed
1tbsp olive oil
2 basil leaves

Making It

1. If you are using fresh tomatoes try and get really ripe ones as they will provide more flavour. Place them in a pot of boiling water for about 30 seconds to get the skins off. If you are using tinned tomatoes they are ready to use.
2. Add all the ingredients to the Nutri Ninja blender cup.
3. Blend for about 20 seconds or until smooth.
4. When ready to eat, heat the sauce up in a saucepan over a low heat for about 10 minutes. You may wish to add a little water to make it a thinner consistency – but only add a little at a time!

Health Benefits

Tomatoes are one of the exceptions when it comes to maintaining, and in this case, increasing, nutritional benefits after cooking. Tomatoes are a fantastic source of lycopene – an antioxidant shown to help prevent certain cancers.

Classic Cheese Sauce

Serves 4

This cheese sauce tastes deliciously smooth, with no lumps! A versatile source that can be poured over cooked vegetables, meat or fish.

Ingredients

460ml milk (semi skimmed milk is fine)
3tbsp butter
3tbsp plain flour
100g grated cheddar cheese

Making It

1. Place the butter in a saucepan and gently melt on a low heat.
2. Turn the heat off and add the flour. Mix well.
3. Gently heat the milk in a saucepan but do not let it boil.
4. Turn a low heat back on the butter and flour mix. Very gradually add the milk in, mixing it well whilst slowly adding more of the milk mixture.
5. Pour the content in to the Nutri Ninja blender. Add the grated cheese and blend until smooth. By putting the cheese sauce through the Nutri Ninja you get rid of any stubborn lumps and are left with a creamy smooth sauce.
6. Serve right away or allow to cool and reheat gently when ready to use.

Health Benefits

Cheddar cheese may be high in calories but it provides essential nutrients including calcium, potassium and protein. Calcium helps maintain your immune system and reduces the risk of osteoporosis.

Spicy Ginger Vinaigrette

A deliciously zingy dressing to drizzle over your favourite salad.

Ingredients

2 garlic cloves, peeled and crushed
Pinch of salt
10g fresh root ginger, grated
4tbps of fresh lemon juice
1tbsp apple cider vinegar
1tbsp curry powder
60ml olive oil

Making It

1.   Place all the ingredients into the Nutri Ninja blender and blend for 20 seconds or until all ingredients are smooth.

Variation: Add 4tbsp mayonnaise and blend for a further 10 seconds and turn it into a dip.

Health Benefits

Fresh ginger adds a delicious warming zing to this dressing. Ginger is well known for its amazing health benefits including acting as a remedy for unsettled stomachs and a decongestant for colds.

Curry powder contains turmeric, a very powerful spice that is said to help a variety of conditions, owing to its anti-inflammatory benefits. It is bright yellow to look at and tastes warm and peppery.

Basil Oil

A really simple dressing to make and drizzle over salads. It also tastes great over roasted tomatoes.

Ingredients

20 fresh basil leaves
1 garlic clove, peeled and crushed
6tbsp extra virgin olive oil

Making It

1.   Add all the ingredients to the Nutri Ninja blender and blend for 10 to 20 seconds or until smooth. Chill in the fridge before serving.

Health Benefits

Basil has high levels of magnesium, vitamins and antioxidants. Magnesium helps with energy levels and has been associated with fighting depression.

Extra virgin olive oil acts as a natural anti-inflammatory, is good for the skin and anti-ageing and strengthens your immune system.

Red Pepper Tomato Sauce

Serves 4

This is a variation on our earlier Simple Pasta Sauce. It goes particularly well with meatballs, pasta, grilled vegetables, or whatever you fancy!

Ingredients

400g tin of chopped tomatoes
1 large onion (approx. 200g)
2 cloves of garlic
1/2 red bell pepper
200ml water
2tbsp brown sugar
2tsp mixed herbs
1tsp salt
1tsp black pepper
1tbsp olive oil
2tbsp apple cider vinegar

Making It

1. Gently heat the olive oil. On a low heat lightly fry the onions for 2 to 3 minutes. Add the crushed garlic cloves and lightly cook for a further 2 to 3 minutes.
2. Add the remaining ingredients and stir. Simmer for around 5 to 10 minutes, or until the tomatoes are soft.
3. Remove from the heat and allow to cool to room temperature.
4. Pour the contents into the Nutri Ninja blender and blend for about 20 seconds or until smooth. If you require a thinner consistency add some warm water and blend again.
5. When you are ready to use the sauce reheat it on a gentle heat for a few minutes.

Health Benefits

Red peppers are low in calories, rich in dietary fibre and also an excellent source of vitamins A, C, and E. Red peppers are a good source of iron so beneficial for people suffering with anaemia.

Mint Sauce

Mint sauce is a tasty accompaniment to lamb. It also works well as a dip. By making it in a blender you get rid of all the mint bits, blending it into a smooth sauce or dip.

Ingredients

30g fresh mint leaves
1tbsp brown sugar
2tbsp apple cider vinegar
150g natural yoghurt (to make a dip)

Making It

1.   Wash the mint leaves and remove the stalks.
2.   If you are making a sauce to use with a lamb joint add all the ingredients into the Nutri Ninja blender apart from the yoghurt and blend until completely smooth.
3.   If you are making a dip, add all the ingredients including the yoghurt to the Nutri Ninja and blend until smooth. Put in the fridge for around 1 hour to allow the mint to infuse with the yoghurt.
4.   Serve with raw vegetables or sliced pitta pockets and dip in!

Health Benefits

Mint is good for digestion and can help sooth stomach inflammations. Mint is also thought to aid weight loss by acting as a stimulant, turning fat into a usable energy.

Jamaican Hot Pepper Sauce

Hot pepper sauce is super tasty splashed on most things – I like to use it as both a dip and as a sauce in burgers or drizzled over chicken and rice.

Ingredients

5 red chilli peppers
400g tomatoes
3 garlic cloves, peeled and crushed
100g finely chopped onions
100ml apple cider vinegar

Making It

1. Put the vinegar into a saucepan and gently cook the chilli peppers in it, for about 3 minutes.
2. Allow to cool and then pour into the Nutri Ninja blender. Add the remaining ingredients. Blend for about 20 to 30 seconds or until smooth.
3. Taste the sauce, if you prefer a hotter sauce, add another chilli pepper!
Note: You can really play around with the heat factor in this recipe. If you prefer a milder taste remove the seeds of the chillies before blending. Alternatively, add more and go for a hotter taste. As always when handling chillies, make sure you wash your hands afterwards.
Variation: Add 100g of ripe mango chunks and blend in to the sauce.

Health Benefits

Red chilli peppers raise endorphin levels, speed up your metabolism and are high in beta-carotene. Studies have shown that red chilli peppers can reduce the cravings of salty, sweet and fatty foods.

Green Pesto

This classic sauce is the perfect accompaniment to stir through a bowl of freshly cooked pasta. Sprinkle some parmesan cheese on top to finish the dish off.

Ingredients

80ml olive oil
40g fresh basil
2 garlic cloves, crushed
60g pine nuts
60g parmesan cheese

Making It

1.   Heat a saucepan for a minute and gently dry fry the pine nuts. Allow to cook for 30 seconds and then toss them over. Cook for a further 30 seconds. Keep on doing this until they just start to go brown. Although you don't have to fry the pine nuts it really helps to release some of their natural oils and taste.

2.   Once the pine nuts have cooled down a little, add them to the Nutri Ninja blender and blend for short bursts of a few seconds at a time. They should be ground down but you may have the odd stubborn pine nut that refuses to be ground! If you are adverse to any crunchy bits in your pasta then remove them now!

3.   Add all the remaining ingredients to the Nutri Ninja blender cup and blend for about 30 seconds or until a smooth paste has been achieved. You may need to keep pausing and scraping the sides down.

4.   Stir into cooked pasta for a tasty, quick meal.

Health Benefits

Pine nuts contain nutrients that can help increase energy levels. They are a good source of magnesium. Pine nuts are also rich in anti-aging antioxidants.

Sweet and Sour Sauce

We love dipping chicken pieces into this sweet and sour sauce, or adding some chunks of pineapple and mixing it with some noodles.

Ingredients

1 red pepper, chopped
1 spring onion, chopped
1 clove garlic, peeled and crushed
Very thin slice of fresh root ginger (4-5mm)
1 can (400g) pineapple chunks in juice
2tbsp cornflour
100g brown sugar
1tbsp soya sauce
3tbsp apple cider vinegar

Making It

1.   Chop the red pepper, spring onion. Peel the garlic clove and put it through a garlic crusher. Slice of a very thin slither of fresh root ginger.
2.   Add 150ml of pineapple juice (from the can) and 100g of pineapple chunks. Leave the remaining pineapple chunks to one side.
3.   Add the red pepper, spring onion, garlic and ginger to the Nutri Ninja blender. Blend for about 20 to 30 seconds or until smooth.
4.   Mix the corn flour with 4tbsp of water in a separate bowl until it has dissolved and there are no lumps. It should have a cream like consistency. Add this to the Nutri Ninja and blend for a further 20 to 30 seconds.
5.   Heat a sauce pan on a high heat and pour the sweet and sour mix into it. Stir in the brown sugar, soya sauce, vinegar and remaining pineapple chunks (if you are just using it as a dip you may want to leave out the pineapple chunks).
6.   Bring to the boil and stir. You will see the sauce quickly get thicker in consistency.
7.   Pour into a dipping bowl or add to your desired dish, it tastes great with stir fried chicken or pork.

Health Benefits

Red peppers are low in calories, rich in dietary fibre and also an excellent source of vitamins A, C, and E. Red peppers are a good source of iron so beneficial for people suffering with anaemia.

Spicy Black Bean Dip

I love the spicy taste to this rich dip. Goes perfectly well with raw vegetable sticks or tortilla chips.

Ingredients

400g tin black eyed beans
Small onion (about 80g), chopped
3 garlic cloves, peeled and crushed
1 jalapeno pepper, seeded and chopped
½ sweet red pepper, chopped
1/3 green pepper, chopped
1tsp ground cumin
1tsp ground chilli powder
2tbsp lime juice
Water (can use water that black eyed beans came in)

Making It

1.   Drain the beans from the tin and reserve the water they came in.
2.   Place all the ingredients in the Nutri Ninja blender and blend for 20 to 30 seconds or until smooth. You may need to keep stopping and scraping the contents from the side of the jar if it gets stuck.
3.   If you find the consistency to thick or lumpy, add some water or the water you reserved from the tin in step 1. Gradually add 1tbsp at a time and blend until you get to your perfect consistency.

Health Benefits

Black eyed beans are a fantastic source of protein, essential for the growth and repair of your body. They are also rich in soluble fibre, helping your body's digestive system. Black eyed beans are high in vitamins A and B. Try and get tinned black eyed beans without added salt. If you can't, rinse them before use.

Cashew Curry Sauce

Serves 4

This sauce is ideal for adding to chicken or a vegetable such as peppers, potatoes or cauliflower and serving with a naan bread and rice.

Ingredients

4 large tomatoes, quartered

3 cloves of garlic, peeled and crushed

1 medium onion (approx. 100g), chopped

2cm fresh root ginger (about 20g), peeled & grated

1tsp ground turmeric

1tsp ground cumin

15 cashew nuts

1tbsp olive oil

1 can coconut milk

Making It

1.   In a large saucepan heat the olive oil. Add the garlic and ginger and gently fry for about 10 seconds.

2.   Add the chopped onion and continue to cook on a gentle heat for a further 2 minutes until the onions are soft.

3.   Add the tomatoes and a pinch of salt and cook until the tomatoes begin to stew, about 15 minutes.

4.   Allow to cool to room temperature and then add to the Nutri Ninja blender. Add the coconut milk, cashew nuts, turmeric and cumin. Blend for about 20 to 30 seconds or until smooth.

5.   Once the contents are smooth return it to the saucepan.

6.   Gently cook on a medium heat until the mix begins to simmer slightly. Turn down the heat as low as it will go and simmer for about 15 minutes, or until the sauce is at your preferred consistency.

7.   Whilst this is simmering cook your chosen meat (or vegetarian option).

8.   Finally, add your meat/vegetables to the sauce and simmer for another 5 minutes taking care not to let the sauce dry out.

Health Benefits

Although cashew nuts are high in calories they are very rich in nutrients and soluble dietary fibre. They are also high in monounsaturated fatty acids, making the nuts heart friendly.

Mango Sauce

Serves 4

This sweet tasting Mango Sauce tastes delicious when combined with stir fried diced chicken breasts and noodles.

Ingredients

100ml chicken stock
1 large orange
1cm fresh root ginger, grated
1 fresh ripe mango, chopped

Making It

1.   Squeeze the juice from the orange. Peel and scoop the flesh out of the mango. The riper the mango is the better.
2.   Place all the ingredients in the Nutri Ninja blender and blend for about 20 to 30 seconds or until smooth.
3.   When you are ready to use the sauce, pour into a sauce pan and cook on a low heat for about 5 to 10 minutes, or until the sauce thickens. Stir in with cooked chicken or noodles.

Health Benefits

Mangoes help boost the body's defences with their high levels of vitamins A and C.

Sweet Chilli Dip

A tasty sauce that can be used for marinating meats in or as a dip for dipping Thai crackers or chicken pieces in.

Ingredients

1tbsp olive oil
3 garlic cloves, peeled and crushed
1tsp tomato puree
250g tomatoes, quartered
3 red chillies
100g dark muscovado sugar
50ml apple cider vinegar

Making It

1.   Prepare the chillies by slicing the tops off and slicing finely. If you like a very mild tasting dip remove all the seeds. If you like a little bit of a chilli after taste leave some or all of the seeds in.
2.   Heat the olive oil on a gentle heat. Add the crushed garlic, tomato puree and cook for about 20 seconds.
3.   Add the tomatoes, sugar, vinegar and chillies. Bring to the boil and allow to boil for about 15 minutes, until the mixture is stodgy.
4.   Switch off the heat and allow the mixture to cool to room temperature.
5.   Pour mixture into the Nutri Ninja and blend for around 20 seconds or until smooth.

Speedy Apple Sauce

I love a generous scoop of apple sauce with my pork. This version can be served raw or if you prefer it a little sweeter, heated up. Either way, it tastes yummy!

Ingredients

1 large apple (Bramley are our favourite)
1tsp fresh lemon juice
1tsp maple syrup
3tbsp water
Pinch of ground cinnamon

Making It

1.   Wash and chop the apples, removing the core.
2.   Add all the ingredients to the Nutri Ninja blender. Start by adding just 3tbsp of water. Blend for a few seconds and stop. Scrape down or any ingredients stuck to the sides (or shake the blender cup). Repeat until you have a puree. Add more water, 1tbsp spoon at a time if you require a thinner consistency.
3.   If you want to eat it warm, heat in a saucepan over a low heat for around 5 minutes. You may need to add a little bit of warm water as required to keep it at the right consistency.

Health Benefits

Bramley apples are rich in dietary fibre, helping to keep your cholesterol levels in check and maintain bowel health.

French Dressing

A classic dressing that goes well with a variety of salads.

Ingredients

8tbsp tomato ketchup
30ml apple cider vinegar
1 small onion, sliced
1tbsp olive oil
½ tsp salt
½ tsp cayenne pepper
½ tsp mustard powder
1tsp paprika
1 garlic clove, peeled and crushed
3tbsp honey
Water (optional)

Making It

1.   Add all the ingredients to the Nutri Ninja blender and blend for 20 to 30 seconds or until smooth. If you require a thinner consistency add some water, 1tbsp at a time.

Health Benefits

Paprika has a distinct taste made from ground peppers. Paprika is rich in iron and potassium as well as being high in vitamin C and carotenoids, providing a variety of health benefits.

Piri Piri Sauce

In Swahili, piri piri means 'pepper pepper.' There are many variations of this sauce. The great thing is you can make it as hot or as mild as you want!

Ingredients

5 red chilli peppers
2 red bell peppers, deseeded
Juice of 1 lemon
4tbsp olive oil
1tbsp ground paprika
2tbsp cayenne pepper
4 cloves garlic, peeled and crushed
1tsp salt

Making It

1. Prepare the chilli peppers by removing the stems and the seeds (if you prefer a hotter sauce leave some or all the seeds in). Deseed the sweet pepper.
2. Add the chilli peppers and all of the remaining ingredients to the Nutri Ninja blender. Blend for about 20 to 30 seconds or until smooth.

Serving Suggestions – use as a marinade for meats, mix in with rice or noodles or just as a tasty dip.

Health Benefits

Red peppers are low in calories, rich in dietary fibre and also an excellent source of vitamins A, C, and E. Red peppers are a good source of iron so beneficial for people suffering with anaemia.

Red chilli peppers raise endorphin levels, speed up your metabolism and are high in beta-carotene. Studies have shown that red chilli peppers can reduce the cravings of salty, sweet and fatty foods.

Bean & Tomato Dip

This dip is not only nutritious, it also tastes great when spread on crackers, oatcakes or breadsticks.

Ingredients

4 tomatoes
2tbsp olive oil
200g cannellini beans, drained
4 garlic cloves, peeled
2tbsp lemon juice
Pinch of pepper

Making It

1. Preheat the oven to 200c (gas mark 6)
2. Quarter the tomatoes and place together with the garlic cloves on a baking tray. Drizzle 1tbsp of olive oil over them. Put in the oven and roast for about 10 to 15 minutes or until they are soft.
3. Remove from the oven and allow to cool slightly.
4. Put everything in the Nutri Ninja blender and blend for about 20 seconds, or until your desired texture is reached.

Health Benefits

Cannellini beans are rich in fibre, low in calories, and high in protein. The soluble fibre content enables you to keep energy levels stable throughout the day and blood sugar levels balanced. Cannellini beans are also a great source of iron.

Tahini Paste

Tahini is conveniently sold in many supermarkets, but what if you could easily make your own?

Ingredients
300g sesame seeds
6tbp light olive oil
Pinch salt (optional)

Making It
1.   Dry fry the sesame seeds on a low heat for about 2 to 3 minutes, taking care not to let them burn. Switch off the heat and allow to cool.
2.   Place the sesame seeds in the Nutri Ninja blender and blend for between 1 and 2 minutes, stopping every 10/20 seconds to shake or scrape the contents from the sides of the blender cup. A crumbly paste should have formed.
3.   Add the olive oil and blend again for a further 2 to 3 minutes, again stopping every 10/20 seconds to shake/scrape the mixture from the sides.
4.   If the mixture is not smooth, add another tbsp. of olive oil and blend again.
5.   Add a pinch of salt to taste (optional) and blend again for a further 10 seconds.
Storage: This can be kept in an airtight container in the fridge for up to 1 month.
Use with our tasty Hummus recipe or our Tomato & Tahini Dip.

Tomato & Tahini Dip

A nutrient rich and easy to make dip. Add a little water to turn it into a tasty salad dressing.

Ingredients
60g sun dried tomatoes
100g (about 7tbsps) tahini
1 garlic clove, peeled and crushed
2tbsp lemon juice
Water (optional, if turning into a salad dressing)

Making It
1.   Add all ingredients to the Nutri Ninja and blend for about 20 to 30 seconds or until smooth.
2.   If you want to use it as a salad dressing add a small amount of water and blend again. Add more water until you reach your desired consistency.

Health Benefits
Tahini paste can be bought in all supermarkets or health food stores. It is made from ground sesame seeds and can be added to a variety of dishes. Nutritional benefits include high levels of iron, calcium, protein and is high in vitamins E, B1, B2, B3, B5 and B15. It is also high in the good fat – unsaturated!
Do you want to make your own tahini? Check out our Tahini Paste to find out how!

Avocado Dip

This guacamole dip has an extra garlicky kick to it. Perfect for dunking raw vegetables in. It also goes well with a bowl full of tortilla crisps!

Ingredients

1 ripe avocado
2 garlic cloves, crushed
1tbsp lemon juice
1tbsp mayonnaise

Making It

1.   Cut the avocado in half and remove the seed. Make sure the avocado is perfectly ripe. Some supermarkets are now selling frozen avocados which are the perfect ripeness and already peeled and destoned. Perfect for keeping on standby in your freezer!

2.   Scoop the flesh out and add to the Nutri Ninja blender. Add the crushed garlic, mayonnaise and lemon juice.

3.   Blend for about 30 seconds or until the dip is at your preferred consistency.

Health Benefits

Avocados are best consumed when they are just ripe. Not only will they taste better, they will also have their full antioxidant benefits or vitamins A, C and E. They are also rich in B vitamins, great for your memory! Avocados are high in fat but it's the good kind – monounsaturated fat.

Hummus

Hummus is the perfect healthy dip. Serve with sliced pitta bread, breadsticks or chopped raw vegetables such as carrots, cucumber and celery.

Ingredients

1 can (400g) chickpeas, drained
2tbsp olive oil
4tbsp fresh lemon juice
2tbsp tahini (see our Tahini Paste if you want to make your own!)
2 garlic cloves, peeled and crushed
Pinch of sea salt
Pinch of cumin
1tsp pepper
Pinch of paprika
60 to 80ml water

Making It

1. Drain the water from the chickpeas.
2. Add all the ingredients to the Nutri Ninja Blender, add the water last but only add about half of it.
3. Blend for 30 seconds, stopping occasionally within this time to scrape the sides down. If the hummus is too thick or not blending properly gradually add some more water. Repeat this process until the mixture is at the perfect consistency.

Health Benefits

Chickpeas are packed with a wide range of health benefits and include high levels or iron, fibre, zinc and copper. Due to the high fibre and protein content of chickpeas they are ideal for helping with weight loss by making you feel fuller for longer whilst consuming less calories.

Tomato Ketchup

Tomato ketchup is a staple condiment in our cupboards. It's great to know what we are putting in this. Feel free to experiment with different spices to change the taste each time you make it. And of course it tastes great with chips!

Ingredients

6 tomatoes
100g dark brown sugar
60ml apple cider vinegar
1tsp mustard powder
1tbsp tomato puree
1tsp Worcestershire sauce
¼ tsp ground coriander
1tsp garlic powder
1 garlic clove, peeled and crushed
¼ tsp all spice
¼ tsp paprika
¼ tsp salt
1tsp cornflour
60ml water

Making It

1.   In a large saucepan mix the apple cider vinegar, garlic powder, paprika, all spice and sugar. Cook on a low heat for 2 to 3 minutes.
2.   Add the remaining ingredients (apart from the cornflour) and simmer on a low heat for about 30 minutes, or until most of the liquid has evaporated and the tomatoes are stewed.
3.   Allow the mixture to cool to room temperature. Add to the Nutri Ninja blender and blend for about 20 seconds, until smooth.
4.   Put the ketchup back into the sauce pan and stir in the cornflour. Simmer for a further 10 minutes.

Storage: Once the ketchup has cooled pour into an airtight container and store in the fridge for up to 1 month.

Health Benefits

Tomatoes are high in antioxidants, which equals great health benefits for you. Tomatoes contain the carotenoids beta-carotene and lycopene. These brightly coloured antioxidants have a vital role in helping to clean up free radicals in the blood system and from body tissues. Antioxidants are also beneficial to slowing down the signs of aging, together with being good for cardiovascular health.

Apple cider vinegar is something that would be great to have in your cupboard. It has so many incredible health benefits, even if you just dilute some with 250ml of water and drink each morning.

Thai Peanut Sauce

A tasty Thai sauce, ideal for dipping chicken kebabs in as a starter, or as part of a main meal.

Ingredients
6tbsp peanut butter
(see our Peanut Butter recipe if you want to make your own!)
1 fresh red chilli, deseeded and chopped
1tbsp lime juice
4tbsp coconut milk
1tbsp fresh root ginger, grated

Making It
1.   Put all the ingredients in the Nutri Ninja blender and blend until smooth, for about 20 seconds.
2.   If you prefer a thicker consistency add 2 to 3tbsp mayonnaise and blend again.

Health Benefits
Peanut butter feels like an indulgent treat, and although it is high in calories (around 94 calories per tablespoon!) it is also rich in health benefits. But, as peanut butter has such a high combination of fibre and protein, you should be left feeling fuller for longer. Peanut butter is packed with vitamin E, magnesium, potassium and vitamin B6.

Of course not all peanut butters are created equal – check the labels before you buy, especially for salt and sugar content. Or better still, make your own! See our Peanut Butter recipe to find out how.

Raspberry Salad Dressing

This raspberry vinaigrette tastes delicious drizzled over a spinach salad. It's quick to make and you can adjust the water content depending on how thick or thin you like it.

Ingredients
60g fresh or frozen raspberries
20ml apple cider vinegar
2tbsp clear honey
1tsp dried basil
80ml olive oil
40ml water

Making It
1. Add all the ingredients to the Nutri Ninja blender, start with just 20ml of water and blend for about 20 seconds. Add more water if you require a thinner consistency.

Health Benefits
Raspberries add a delicious sweet taste to this salad dressing. Raspberries are packed with nutrients and are low in fat and calories. They are rich in fibre and antioxidants such as vitamin C.

Creamy Jalapeno Dip

A delicious dip that can be made as hot as you can handle. Goes perfect with tortilla crisps or crunchy raw vegetables.

Ingredients

½ tbsp. olive oil
½ jalapeno pepper, chopped
2 garlic cloves, peeled and crushed
125g cream cheese
½ medium tomato
½ small red pepper
½ tsp paprika

Making It

1.   Prepare the jalapeno according to how hot (spicy) you want your dip. If you want a milder taste remove the seeds and membrane. If you like it hotter, leave some or all of them in.
2.   Heat the olive oil on a gentle heat in a saucepan. Add the crushed garlic and sliced jalapeno pepper. Cook on a gentle heat for about 2 minutes.
3.   Allow to cool and then add to the Nutri Ninja blender together with the other ingredients. Blend for 20 to 30 seconds or until smooth.

Health Benefits

Jalapeno peppers are low in calories and high in vitamins C and A. The capsaicin in jalapeno peppers can potentially help with weight loss by increasing your metabolic rate.

CURRY PASTES

Curry pastes are really easy to make in the Nutri Ninja. The power of the motor means that the ingredients mix really effectively to form the paste.

The ingredients can be doubled, or even tripled, to freeze portions to use another time.

You might find that your blender cup requires a deep clean after you've made a curry paste. I tend to use the juice of a lemon mixed in with some water and just switch the blender on to whizz it around. You can also use vinegar or baking soda mixed in with some water.

Thai Red Curry Paste

This Thai Red Curry paste is really easy to make and can be used as a base for curries, stir fry dishes and soups. It's worth making this much so you can keep some in the freezer and defrost it when you want it. By making your own paste you can adjust the hot factor!

Ingredients

6 garlic cloves, peeled
3 inches (approx. 70g) fresh root ginger, sliced

2tbsp black pepper
2tbsp tomato puree
5 whole red chillies, chopped
50g lemongrass, chopped
100g onion, chopped
40g fresh coriander leaves

5tbsp chilli garlic sauce
1tbsp ground coriander
1tbsp ground cumin
Pinch salt
Juice & zest of 1 lime

Making It

1.   Peel the garlic cloves and slice the fresh root ginger. Chop the lemongrass and onion. Chop the red chilli into slices – if you like your Thai dishes very hot leave the seeds in. If you like it medium leave half in. If you like it milder, remove them all.
2.   Grate the lime skin to create a zest. Add all the other ingredients to the Nutri Ninja blender and then squeeze the juice from the lime in as well.
3.   Blend for 10 seconds and shake the blender cup, repeat until a paste has formed.
4.   You can now use this with stir fried diced chicken or beef. Mix in a can of coconut milk to make a tasty Thai Red Curry.

Health Benefits

This paste contains a wide range of health benefits.

The coriander contains many essential vitamins and minerals, including iron.

Garlic is very nutritious, in particular because of the sulfur compound, allicin.

Cumin, a spice popular in many world cuisines is useful for digestion, the immune system, anaemia amongst many other benefits. Lemongrass is a popular herb used in Asian dishes, the plant contains multiple antioxidants and has many potential health benefits, including lowering cholesterol.

Tikka Paste

A mild curry, especially popular in the UK! This paste is perfect for making chicken tikka masala.

Ingredients

2tbsp ground almonds
1 red chilli, deseeded
1tsp ground cumin
¾ tsp ground coriander
2 garlic cloves
2cm ginger root (10-15g)
1tsp garam masala
½ tsp sea salt
2tbsp olive oil
1tbsp tomato puree
3tbsp desiccated coconut
20ml water

Making It

1.   Remove the seeds from the red chilli and then place all the ingredients in the Nutri Ninja blender.

2.   Blend for about 20 seconds, scrape down the contents from the side and blend again for a further 20 seconds. Continue to do this until a smooth paste has formed. Serving Suggestion – Heat 1tbsp of vegetable oil in a saucepan, add a medium chopped onion and cook for a few minutes until golden. Add the chicken tikka paste and cook for a further 3 minutes. Add 500g of diced chicken breast and cook until the meat is sealed. Add 400g of chopped tomatoes and 100ml of water and simmer for around 5 minutes. Add 150g of double cream and stir in, simmer for a further 10 minutes until the sauce has thickened and the chicken is cooked through. Serve with rice and naan bread.

Tandoori Paste

A popular Indian paste to add to both chicken and fish dishes.

Ingredients

24 garlic cloves, peeled and crushed
5cm fresh root ginger, chopped
3tbsp coriander seeds (or 2tbsp of ground coriander)
3tbsp cumin seeds (or 2tbsp of ground cumin)
3tbsp ground fenugreek
3tbsp ground paprika
3 red chillies
3tbsp English mustard (or 2tbsp of English mustard powder)
2tbsp tomato puree
1tsp salt
8tbsp water

Making It

1. Slice the red chillies up and de-seed them unless you want to have a very hot tandoori.
2. Add all the ingredients to the Nutri Ninja blender and blend for about 2 – 3 minutes, stopping occasionally to scrape the sides to ensure it is fully blended. Continue until a paste has been formed. If the paste is too thick, then you may need to add another couple of tablespoons of water to loosen it up while blending.

Serving Suggestion

Use about half of the mixture to make your chicken or fish dish (add yoghurt, oil & lemon juice to the paste and marinate the meat in it for around 5 hours before cooking).

Health Benefits

Fenugreek is rich in many minerals including iron, potassium, selenium, copper, zinc, manganese, magnesium and calcium.

There is A LOT of garlic in this recipe! Garlic is very nutritious, in particular because of the sulfur compound, allicin. Allicin is known to have great anti-viral, anti-fungal, anti-bacterial and anti-oxidant properties. Garlic is thought to lower blood pressure as well as being a fantastic source of manganese, selenium, vitamin C, B6 and a selection of minerals.

SPREADS & BUTTERS

You can really use your imagination when it comes to creating new spreads and butters.

When we first tried a chocolate spread in our Nutri Ninja I didn't think we would be able to get a smooth enough texture. I was also concerned that the blender would give up with all that extra work to do! You just need to keep on blending, making sure you stop every so often, then blend again. It will eventually turn to a buttery spread and is well worth the extra blending time! Our Nutri Ninja has stood up to many batches of nut butters using this method.

Chocolate Spread

We LOVE Nutella in our house. It was inevitable that we wouldn't be long before we replicated it with our own homemade version! Delicious.

Ingredients

170g toasted hazelnuts
1 tbsp coconut oil (optional)
30g cocoa powder
1 tsp vanilla extract
75g maple syrup

Making It

1.   Preheat the oven to 180C. Spread the hazelnuts out on a baking tray and put in the oven for about 10 to 15 minutes or until the skins start go a little black.
2.   Once they have cooled down a little place them on a damp kitchen tea towel and spread them out. Fold the kitchen towel over and vigorously rub the hazelnuts. This is to try and remove as much of the skin as you can.
3.   Pick the hazelnuts out and place them in the cup of the Nutri Ninja. Add the cocoa powder, vanilla extract, maple syrup and coconut oil (if using). Start to blend for a short burst at a time (about 10 seconds). Continue to do this for around 2 to 3 minutes until the mixture is smooth. You may need to stop and use a knife to scrape the mixture down from the sides.

Continue to blend in short bursts, stopping when you need to scrape the mixture from the sides.

4.   Do a taste test. If you prefer a sweeter taste add more maple syrup.

Please note: Although this is very yummy indeed, it won't be exactly like the shop bought version. But remember, you know all the ingredients you have put in to create your very own healthy version!

Storage: Keep in an airtight container in the fridge for up to 7 days.

Health Benefits

The high Vitamin E content of hazelnuts make them great for your skin and maintaining a healthy blood supply. They are also an excellent source of protein, calcium, magnesium, fibre and other minerals. They are also high in healthy unsaturated fat making them heart friendly.

Maple Syrup is a great alternative to sugar. It also has less calories than honey, another popular sugar substitute. Maple syrup also has numerous antioxidant properties that are essential for a healthy lifestyle.

Cocoa powder is a great way to satisfy your chocolate craving, without feeling guilty. Cocoa powder is high in antioxidants, fibre, iron and magnesium. It is also thought that cocoa might be able to increase endorphins. Try to go for a raw cocoa powder which will be less processed and keep more health benefits.

Peanut Butter

I adore peanut butter. I can quite happily eat it by the spoonful. It was for this reason I knew I needed to find a healthy version!

Ingredients

200g unsalted peanuts
1tbsp honey
1tsp salt (optional)
1tbsp coconut oil (optional)

Making It

1. Dry fry the peanuts in a frying pan or saucepan for about 5 minutes. Do not allow to burn.
2. Place them in the Nutri Ninja blender with the honey and blend for short bursts of a few seconds at a time, until grounded. Scrape the sides down. Please be advised that the manufacturers advise not to use dry ingredients without liquid in the Nutri Ninja blender. Although we have successfully made this recipe without any problems, please do refer to the manual that came with your blender if in doubt.
3. Keep on with this process for around 2 to 3 minutes. Keep on stopping to scrape/shake the contents. All of a sudden the mixture will turn into a smooth buttery spread. Keep going until you get to this stage. If the peanuts are struggling to form a paste, add 1tbsp of coconut oil and blend again.
4. If after tasting the peanut butter you prefer a sweeter and/or saltier taste, add the salt and 1tbsp honey and blend again.

Storage: Put in an airtight container in the fridge. Use within 7 days.

Alternatives: Substitute the peanuts for another nut of your choice; cashews or almonds also work really well when turning into a nut butter.

Health Benefits

Peanuts are a fantastic healthy energy source. They are rich in vitamins, anti-oxidants, nutrients and minerals. The mono-unsaturated fatty acids in peanuts can increase good cholesterol in the body. The high level of proteins present are essential for promoting the healthy growth and development of the body.

Mixed Nut Butter

A slight variation on the popular peanut butter. Mix in some more nuts for added taste and additional health benefits. This tastes soooo good. I love dipping crunchy apple slices in it!

Ingredients

200g mixed unsalted nuts (cashew, almonds, peanuts, hazelnuts, whatever you can get)

Pinch of salt (optional)

1tsp honey (optional)

Making It

1.   Dry fry the nuts in a frying pan or saucepan for about 5 minutes. Do not allow to burn.

2.   Place them in the Nutri Ninja blender with the honey and blend for short bursts of a few seconds at a time, until grounded. Scrape the sides down. Please be advised that the manufacturers advise not to use dry ingredients without liquid in the Nutri Ninja blender. Although we have successfully made this recipe without any problems, please do refer to the manual that came with your blender if in doubt.

3.   Keep on with this process for around 2 to 3 minutes. Keep on stopping to scrape/shake the contents. All of a sudden the mixture will turn into a smooth buttery spread. Keep going until you get to this stage.

4.   The next bit is optional. I quite like it with just nuts and honey but some people might like the pinch of salt to give it that store bought taste. Add the salt and more honey if required and blend again. Do a taste test and add more or either according to how you like it.

Storage: Put in an airtight container in the fridge. Use within 7 days.

Health Benefits

Nuts are sometimes avoided because of the high calories and fat content found within them. But the fats are unsaturated and a handful of mixed nuts are a real nutrient powerhouse. Nuts contain so much protein that fills you up for longer, so you can satisfy those cravings.

It's worth trying to put in some walnuts as they have the highest level of omega-3 fatty acids.

Cashew nuts are very rich in iron and zinc, great for anaemia, healthy skin and as an immune system booster.

Brazil nuts are another powerful nut to include, just a few will provide your body with all the selenium your body needs. Selenium is a very powerful antioxidant needed for good eyesight, healthy skin and hair and healthy muscles, including heart muscles.

Chocco Coco Almond Spread

This spread tastes great on apples, strawberries or spread on a tortilla wrap and heated up.

Ingredients

220g roasted almonds
2tbsp cocoa powder
3tbsp coconut oil
Pinch of salt (optional)

Making It

1.   Add the almonds, coconut oil and cocoa powder to the Nutri Ninja blender and blend for 2 to 3 minutes, stopping every 10/20 seconds to scrape the sides down or shake the mixture. Keeping repeating this process until you have a creamy mixture.
2.   Taste the butter. Add a pinch of salt if desired and blend again.

Storage: Put in an airtight container in the fridge. Use within 7 days.

Health Benefits

Almonds are full of healthy fats. It is preferable to use unsalted roasted almonds and add salt as required. However, if you are unable to get hold of the unsalted variety then just don't add any extra salt. Almonds are rich in fibre, protein, vitamin E and magnesium. Vitamin E helps to keep your skin looking young and maintain a healthy blood supply.

CPSIA information can be obtained
at www.ICGtesting.com
Printed in the USA
BVHW090753070821
613846BV00006B/719